THE BETTER BRAIN

THE
BETTER BRAIN

Overcome Anxiety, Combat Depression, and Reduce ADHD and Stress with Nutrition

BONNIE J. KAPLAN, PhD

JULIA J. RUCKLIDGE, PhD

HOUGHTON MIFFLIN HARCOURT

Boston • New York

2021

For information about permission to reproduce selections from this book,
write to trade.permissions@hmhco.com or to Permissions,
Houghton Mifflin Harcourt Publishing Company, 3 Park Avenue,
19th Floor, New York, New York 10016.

hmhbooks.com

Library of Congress Cataloging-in-Publication Data
Names: Kaplan, Bonnie J., author. | Rucklidge, Julia J., author.
Title: The better brain : overcome anxiety, combat depression, and reduce
ADHD and stress with nutrition / Bonnie J. Kaplan, PhD, Julia J. Rucklidge, PhD.
Description: Boston : Houghton Mifflin Harcourt, 2021. |
Includes bibliographical references and index.
Identifiers: LCCN 2020039114 (print) | LCCN 2020039115 (ebook) |
ISBN 9780358447108 (hardcover) | ISBN 9780358449263 |
ISBN 9780358449447 | ISBN 9780358447085 (ebook)
Subjects: LCSH: Mental illness — Nutritional aspects. |
Mental illness — Diet therapy.
Classification: LCC RC455.4.N8 K37 2021 (print) | LCC RC455.4.N8 (ebook) |
DDC 616.85/270654 — dc23
LC record available at https://lccn.loc.gov/2020039114
LC ebook record available at https://lccn.loc.gov/2020039115

Book design by Chloe Foster
Infographics rendered by Mapping Specialists, Ltd.

Printed in the United States of America
DOC 10 9 8 7 6 5 4 3 2 1

This book presents, among other things, the research and ideas of its authors. It is not intended to be a substitute for consultation with a professional healthcare practitioner. Consult with your healthcare practitioner before starting any diet or other medical regimen. The publisher and the author disclaim responsibility for any adverse effects resulting directly or indirectly from information contained in this book. Some names and identifying details have been changed.

To all our research participants, who give us their time and trust, and to our graduate students and trainees, who will carry this work forward into the future.

CONTENTS

PART III

HOW TO FEED YOUR BRAIN

FOREWORD

by Andrew Weil, MD

New York Times best-selling author of *Spontaneous Happiness* and director of the University of Arizona Center for Integrative Medicine

IN MY FOUR YEARS (1964–68) as a student at Harvard Medical School, the total instruction I received in nutrition was thirty minutes during a clinical rotation — grudgingly allowed for a hospital dietitian to talk about special diets available to patients. That deficiency in medical education persists, although — finally — it is recognized as a problem.[1] Because most physicians are not nutritionally literate, they tend not to understand the influence of dietary choices on health status and disease risks or the power of dietary change as a primary therapeutic strategy.

These subjects are key components of Integrative Medicine training and practice for dealing with physical illnesses. When I write treatment plans for patients, almost always the first items are recommendations for dietary modification; often, I find these alone to be sufficient. Combined with other lifestyle changes, natural remedies, and mind/body therapies, they may obviate the need for medication or, if medication is necessary, make it possible to use lower doses of less potent agents.

In cases of autoimmunity, for example, adopting an anti-inflammatory diet and supplementing it with omega-3 fatty acids (from fish oil or other sources) and natural anti-inflammatory agents like turmeric and ginger may reduce symptoms significantly. Together with mindfulness and stress management training and, possibly, traditional Chinese medicine, improvement may be so great that need for immunosuppressive drugs is much less. For managing gastro-esophageal reflux disease, instead of resorting immediately to proton pump inhibitors with all of their serious short- and long-term adverse effects, integrative practitioners can take dietary histories and advise patients about eliminating common irritants (like coffee and decaffeinated coffee), changing the timing and size of meals, managing stress, and experimenting with safe natural products like chamomile, DGL (deglycyrrhizinated licorice), and d-limonene.

Given the relevance of nutrition to health and the safety and efficacy of dietary modification for the management of diverse ailments, why have these subjects so consistently been neglected in the training of physicians? The only explanation I come up with is that to the academic medical mind, nutrition looks more like home economics than "real" science. Whatever the reason, the consequences are detrimental, limiting understanding of the causes of disease and options for treatment and contributing to overuse of medications.

Further, deficiency of education in nutrition has skewed research priorities. In the past few years, a flood of much-publicized studies — many of them poorly designed meta-analyses — have belittled the benefits and exaggerated the dangers of dietary supplements, particularly multinutrient products.[2] Medical journals have given these reports prominence, leading to stories in the popular media suggesting that people taking vitamin and mineral supplements are not only wasting their money but are also increasing their risks of all-cause mortality. One can speculate about the motivations for this agenda, but its influence is clear: despite evidence to the contrary, many clinicians now advise patients not to use these supplements.

Neglect of nutrition and of dietary supplementation is a serious defect in medicine generally and in the field of mental health particularly. The biomedical paradigm that dominates that field explains all mental and emotional disorders as the result of disordered brain biochemistry and relies almost exclusively on psychiatric medication to manage them. The limitations of that paradigm should be obvious: despite very high rates of prescribing those drugs, the conditions they are supposed to treat, such as depression and anxiety, remain epidemic in society. Their efficacy is unimpressive and their adverse effects significant. In long-term use, they may actually prolong or worsen the problems they are meant to relieve.[3]

The field of integrative mental health is in its infancy, but given the inadequacy of the pharmaceutical approach, it is attracting growing numbers of mental health professionals. Nutrition is an important focus of the field, with due attention to dietary change as a primary treatment strategy along with appropriate use of micronutrient supplementation.

The authors of this book have been studying nutrition and brain health for years. Their research provides strong evidence for dietary adjustment and supplementation as safe and effective ways to optimize mental health and treat the most common mental and emotional disorders. Yet Bonnie Kaplan and Julia Rucklidge write, "We both had been taught that nutrition and diet were of trivial significance for mental health, and that only drugs or psychotherapy were of any value as treatments." In these pages, they explain how they came to question that dogma and begin their groundbreaking studies. They also discuss the opposition they encountered to their recommendations for multinutrient rather than single-nutrient supplementation.

In recent years, other lines of research have added to our understanding of the relationship between what people eat and cognitive and emotional status. Two discoveries I consider especially noteworthy are the connection between inflammation and depression and the interactions of the gut microbiome with the brain, both of which are explained in this book.

The rationale for reliance on the most commonly prescribed antidepressant medications (selective serotonin reuptake inhibitors) is the assumption that depression results from deficiency of serotonin at neural junctions in the brain. If this were the whole story, one would expect drugs that increase serotonin at those junctions to be more effective than they are. In fact, the more we study SSRIs, the harder it is to distinguish their effects from those of placebos, except in the most severe forms of depression.

An alternative concept — the cytokine hypothesis of depression — posits a correlation between the immune system and the brain: specifically, that upregulation of inflammatory cytokines is linked to depressed mood and the various symptoms that often accompany it, such as fatigue, decreased appetite, and social withdrawal. This suggests that moderating inflammation can help prevent and treat depression and benefit emotional well-being. One way to do that is to adopt an anti-inflammatory diet.

The mainstream North American diet is clearly pro-inflammatory. It provides fats and forms of carbohydrates that favor inflammation and not enough of the protective elements found in vegetables, fruits, herbs, spices (notably turmeric and ginger), and beverages like green tea. Using the Mediterranean diet as a reference point, Drs. Kaplan and Rucklidge discuss the importance of food choices to keep excessive inflammation in check and optimize brain health. They advise what and what not to eat and even provide easy-to-follow recipes.

Understanding of the influence of the gut microbiome on brain function has developed even more recently. As a medical student, all I learned about gut flora was that they played a role in digestion. Back then, no one suspected that the microorganisms in the gastrointestinal tract affected general health, our interactions with the environment, or the brain. Now we know those organisms produce neurotransmitters and other regulatory compounds, some of which travel to centers in the brain by way of the vagus nerve. Remarkably, the composition and activities of the gut microbiome appear to be factors in autism, ADHD, mood disorders, and

Parkinson's disease. The more diverse the microbial population of the gastrointestinal tract, the better, especially with a preponderance of bacterial species known to be associated with better health. Dietary patterns strongly influence which microorganisms thrive in the gut and which do not. That subject is also covered in these pages.

In presenting this material and summarizing their own research, Drs. Kaplan and Rucklidge say they are giving us a "bold new paradigm" of mental health. I congratulate them for it. Making nutritional science central to the field is long overdue. It promises safer and more effective ways to prevent and treat mental and emotional disorders and suggests simple, practical steps that all of us can take to optimize brain health. I could not be more pleased to introduce it to readers.

Cortes Island, British Columbia, Canada

July 2020

INTRODUCTION

Finding Answers in Nutrition, Not the Pharmacy

THERE IS AN ENORMOUS crisis in America right now. Not just an economic crisis or an obesity crisis or an opioid crisis. A *mental health* crisis.

Currently, *one person in every five* has some form of mental health issue. This is incredibly disturbing, because a mental health challenge in one individual affects an entire family, which means that the number affected is much higher.

Yet for over fifty years, modern medicine has been trying — mostly unsuccessfully — to treat mental disorders with pharmaceuticals. For example:

- All indicators across all Western countries show that mood and anxiety disorders have not decreased over the last few decades — actually, they've *gone way up* — despite substantial increases in the prescriptions of medications, particularly antidepressants. Right now about 40 million Americans take some kind of psychiatric medication: that's equivalent to about one in six adults.[1] According to an article published in the *New York Times* on April 7, 2018, 15.5 million Americans have been taking antidepressants in particular for at least five years. This rate has almost doubled since 2010, and more than tripled since 2000.

- Despite an ever-increasing use of antidepressants, recovery rates and relapse rates aren't any better now than they were fifty years ago before the advent of medications.
- According to the CDC (Centers for Disease Control), suicide rates in the United States have increased steadily from 2000 to 2016.

Conventional treatment helps some, but doesn't solve the problem. Many people remain shamed by the unfair social stigma around mental health issues, putting them at risk for even worse symptoms of depression and anxiety.

In addition, the impact on healthcare budgets of these often ineffective treatments *is huge*. It costs the US economy tens of billions of dollars for treatments that just aren't working well enough. Not to mention the cost to consumers who can't afford insurance or copays.

What if there *is* a solution to this crisis?

What if the pharmaceuticals that are costly, ineffective for many, and laden with side effects were no longer the automatic go-to treatment for mental health issues?

What if we could eliminate that social stigma by showing that many mental health symptoms in some people are simply caused by suboptimal nutrition and not by something being "wrong" with you?

What if the right nutritional approach to treating mental health issues can save as much as 90 percent of society's mental healthcare budget?

What if one solution to this crisis is as simple as changing how you eat?

Nutrition matters, much more than you may realize. We all know that eating poorly can cause all kinds of physical illnesses, like obesity, Type II diabetes, cardiovascular disease, and premature death. But poor nutrition is also a significant risk factor for the development of *mental* illness.

Why? Because when we eat, most of the energy and nutrients we consume are used by our brains. What you eat today will affect how you feel and think tomorrow. Most people don't know that. They might think that a healthy diet is needed for overall health, but not realize its importance for better mental health.

The Better Brain is the first book that will tell you how and why nutrients can be used to treat mental health issues. We are scientists who've shown that many symptoms of anxiety, depression, attention deficit/hyperactivity disorder (ADHD), post-traumatic stress disorder (PTSD), and more are caused by suboptimal nutrition.

In other words, what if a large part of the solution to this mental health crisis is as simple as changing what you feed your brain?

This book is all about that solution.

How This Book Came to Be

With medication I got better — with the nutrients I got *normal.*
— AUTUMN STRINGAM

After her first baby was born in 1992, a Canadian woman named Autumn Stringam had such a severe postpartum psychosis that she was admitted to the psychiatric ward at the University of Alberta in Edmonton. On the fateful day in late 1996 that Bonnie met her, along with her father Tony Stephan (a property manager) and their friend David Hardy (a nutrition consultant and feed formulator for farm animals), she described the auditory and visual hallucinations that she had had; the five psychiatric medications she was required to take; the fact that she was not permitted to be alone with her baby in case the voices in her head returned and told her again to kill her baby; her doctors' prognosis that she would never be well; and her determination to do whatever her doctors told her so that maybe she could have a better life.

And then she told Bonnie what happened when she took a broad spectrum of micronutrients — the term we use for minerals and vitamins —

as recommended by her father and David. She began to feel well, like herself again. She was able to gradually eliminate her medications. Her hallucinations disappeared.

And her psychiatrist threatened to stop seeing her if she continued with micronutrients instead of medications.

Autumn's family, the Stephans, had several members suffering from bipolar disorder, psychosis, and depression — serious mental health issues. Conventional treatment did not restore them to normal mental health, and there were many challenging side effects and constant relapses. In desperation, and supported by David Hardy's nutrition knowledge, along with Tony's children and others, they began using over-the-counter pills and liquids containing micronutrients. Much to everyone's surprise, they got better. A *lot* better!

The idea of using micronutrients to improve emotional stability was well established in animals used in laboratory research, and in the 1990s supplemental micronutrients were used in farm animals across Alberta. In humans, the pioneering work of Saskatchewan-based Dr. Abram Hoffer in the 1950s showed clinical benefits in people given large doses of niacin, later leading to a strong orthomolecular community in Canada, which continues to this day to focus on nutritional treatments of mental health problems.

When Tony Stephan's children improved sufficiently to be able to function normally without psychiatric medication, Tony and his friend David anticipated great interest within the psychiatric and scientific community. To attract the attention of a local academic neuroscientist, Bryan Kolb, David and Tony collected data from some friends whose children had ADHD and emotional outbursts. Dr. Kolb analyzed the data and sent the results to Bonnie in August 1996, because he knew she had published on nutrition in the past.

Shocked yet intrigued, Bonnie knew she had to investigate this further . . . and that was what started her, and soon Julia, on the improbable path toward upending conventional beliefs about the treatment of mental illness.

A dual American/Canadian citizen who earned her academic degrees in America as an experimental psychologist, with postdoctoral training in neurophysiology, Bonnie had been working as a professor in the Department of Pediatrics at the University of Calgary in 1993, studying neurodevelopmental disorders (such as dyslexia and ADHD), when Julia started her PhD under her supervision while also training to become a clinical psychologist. Like all students of psychology, and like all medical students at the time, we both had been taught that nutrition and diet were of trivial significance for mental health, and that only drugs or psychotherapy were of any value as treatments.

After Julia earned her doctorate in 1998 (based on research looking at the psychosocial outcomes of women with ADHD), she moved first to Toronto for postdoctoral training at the Hospital for Sick Children and then in 2000 to New Zealand for an academic post at the University of Canterbury. She stayed in touch with Bonnie, who continued to study the biological basis of learning and attention problems. Bonnie's postdoctoral training in neurophysiology and her work in behavior genetics generated her interest in the underlying physiology behind human behavior and mental health, and along with some of her Canadian colleagues, she started studying the effect on mental health of the micronutrients used by Autumn. Bonnie began publishing data in 2001, with results showing that with micronutrients, these people not only got well, but *stayed* well, and with none of the horrible side effects that commonly occurred with psychiatric meds.

After Julia nominated her for a visiting fellowship in New Zealand, Bonnie went to the University of Canterbury in 2003 to teach about the role of nutrition in mental health. When she presented her preliminary data, Julia was fascinated — but it was both the remarkable turnaround for people who were so severely ill and the replications observed across a number of different scientists and clinicians that really gained Julia's attention.

From Julia's perspective — based on her own work and that of many others around the world — conventional treatments were not making enough people well. It is the role of scientists to be the critic and conscience of society. It's also our role to investigate new ideas, no matter how controversial, and no matter how much the idea might contravene the current way of thinking. So Julia thought, what do we have to lose? We either discover these micronutrients aren't helpful, which the public might like to know; or we find out they *are* helpful, which both the government and the public really should know.

Julia began to publish the results of her own studies starting in 2009. And she observed exactly what Bonnie had seen already: *micronutrients worked.* Her first case was a teenager with OCD (obsessive-compulsive disorder) whom she had been treating for over a year with CBT (cognitive behavior therapy) with minimal change. He went on the micronutrients, and within a week, his symptoms had virtually disappeared. She observed others showing dramatic improvements. The micronutrients helped many people recover from what seemed like intractable and chronic conditions.

Both of us continued to study the role of micronutrients and brain health, Bonnie at the University of Calgary in Canada, and Julia at the Mental Health and Nutrition Research lab at the University of Canterbury in Christchurch, New Zealand.

Broad-Spectrum Multinutrients

Our research never would have come to be without the astonishing discovery by Tony Stephan and David Hardy in southern Alberta. At the time, they knew that mainstream medical practitioners considered only two nutritional options when trying to correct brain dysfunction: treatment with a single nutrient at a time (the way nutritional research had been conducted since the 1920s), or treatment with a select favorite-few nutrients (the way many clinicians approach mental health even now). Tony and David's breakthrough — which in hindsight seems so obvious! — was their decision to provide *all the major minerals and vitamins together, in balance, at appropriate doses,* in one supplement, which we will refer to as broad-spectrum <u>multi</u>nutrients.

They only had to look at Autumn for proof, as she hasn't needed any psychiatric medication since she started taking micronutrient supplements in 1996.

After that eureka moment, Tony and David quit their jobs and formed the first company, Truehope Nutritional Support, to manufacture a broad-spectrum multinutrient formula — meaning that it contained thirty or so dietary minerals and vitamins, along with some amino acids and antioxidants. It was initially called EMPower; over the years small modifications resulted in amendments to the name (EMPowerplus, EMPowerplus Advanced). We refer to it in this book as **EMP.**

After working together for about fifteen years, David and Tony completed a planned business separation, where David started an independent company, Hardy Nutritionals. Their supplement, Daily Essential Nutrients, is very similar, containing the full spectrum of essential minerals and vitamins. We refer to it throughout as **DEN.**

With this kind of broad-spectrum supplement in hand, Bonnie and Julia, as well as additional scientists, finally had reliable products to use in their research. Because EMP and DEN have been studied in academic settings in three countries, the government health regulators in all those countries have examined and approved the formulas for research. That approval affirms the quality and stability of the ingredients, which is required by university research ethics committees. EMP and DEN have been the subject of more than fifty peer-reviewed publications ever since.

Have you ever felt frustrated when you read "vitamin D is good for depression" followed by "vitamin D has no effect on depression"? So often, the science is inconsistent because the studies used different formulations and different doses. This is why there is such a huge advantage in having a reliable product used for multiple studies, scrutinized by governments for the ingredient sources, purity, quality, and stability. Now, with the Alberta formulas, scientists around the globe have a way to study the full spectrum of micronutrients that every brain requires, and a way to compare their findings and replicate each other's work. The result: a clear message is provided for the public — and now, for you, in this book!

On the other hand, there is nothing in this research that says that *only* EMP and DEN benefit mental health. What both David and Tony taught the researchers was that we'd all benefit from having *more* high-quality formulas for independent scientists to study. These two families didn't go into business to monopolize the field or to scam consumers, but to help them; their goal is to change the way people with mental health problems are treated, and to give them an alternative to prescription meds. When Tony and David realized that psychiatrists would rarely support patients desperately trying to decrease or get off psychiatric meds that had given them debilitating side effects, they set up telephone lines with product specialists to help people who wanted to try broad-spectrum multinutrients. We know of no other natural health product companies that have chosen to focus on developing this kind of product for mental health or support for families.

What Is Micro and What Is Multi When Referring to Nutrients?

In chapter 2 we will provide some standard definitions of nutrients, vitamins, and minerals. But in the meantime, we need to clarify the use of two terms used throughout the book. *Micronutrient* in general refers to minerals or vitamins or both together. But as you will see, the two of us have done quite a few studies of some products that contain lots of micronutrients, and sometimes a few other things in addition—such as amino acids. How can we talk to you about a formula containing around thirty micronutrients alongside other nutrients in a way that specifies its breadth? We have settled on the term *broad-spectrum multinutrient formula*, or just *multinutrient formula*, to indicate that it contains lots of nutrients.

Why Don't You Know About This Powerful Treatment?

Does the mental health world celebrate these multinutrient companies? No, it does not. Instead, it is highly suspicious and dismissive. Mental health clinicians have been slow to acknowledge *any* published scientific research on *any* aspect of nutrition's role in mental health, not just the fifty peer-reviewed publications on EMP and DEN.

We should consider three reasons for this selective dismissal of nutrition:

• *The first reason* is the inadequacy of nutrition education (discussed in chapter 1). Bonnie used to end lectures on her early research with the following topic: "Why it all makes sense." She did so because twenty years ago, people seemed to think that resolving mental health problems with nutrients was very close to magical thinking. Western society had been taught to focus on eating a healthy diet to have strong muscles and bones (obviously important), while not being taught to feed their brains (discussed in chapter 2). Sadly, years of funded research devoted to manipulating a single nutrient at a time — what we call magic bullet thinking — has also contributed to the impression that vitamins and minerals are trivial factors in brain health.

Education for our physicians is a particular problem, as it is often delivered directly or indirectly from pharmaceutical companies. And the scientific research is too. When Bonnie was trained in the 1960s and 1970s, no scientist with integrity would *ever* take money from any company. It's almost comical to remember those days! Now pharmaceutical companies are the major financial driver of all clinical trials in mental health, leading to an era of misrepresentation of the efficacy and safety of meds.[2] Chapter 1 reviews other ways in which the information about safe and efficacious treatments has been skewed by pharmaceutical funds.

For this reason, we have chosen to have absolutely *no financial ties* to any supplement company. From the beginning of our research on EMP, DEN, and other nutrients described in this book, we decided to go back to the good old days. We have *no* commercial ties and *no* conflicts of interest.

Who benefits from misleading the public? For one, the pharmaceutical companies who make psychiatric medications. And the supplement companies selling their single-nutrient formulas, which may not be bad, but aren't good enough to resolve mental health challenges, as we'll explain. People buy a bottle of a single vitamin or two, try them, are disappointed, and this failure usually leads them back to the psychiatric meds they were desperate to stop taking in the first place.

We hear about this desperation all the time. People come to us for advice because we have written extensively on this topic in scientific journals as well as through blogs and newspaper articles, and we have spoken publicly even more about how vitamins and minerals and better nutrition improve mental health. We've also both given hundreds of lectures all over the world at universities, at conferences, and to the public. In October 2014, Julia gave a TEDx Talk on "The Surprisingly Dramatic Role of Nutrition in Mental Health" and it has since gotten over 1.6 million views on YouTube. It's proof of how strongly our message resonates with the public.

Since we've been working together, time and again, in lectures to audiences ranging from 25 to 1,200, we've asked the listeners to raise their hands if they or people close to them were struggling with mental health challenges. The response has always been close to 100 percent — which in itself is shocking. Then we ask: "Please raise your hands again if the people you're thinking of have found that conventional treatments resolved their problems." Almost always, not a single hand is raised. One time, when Bonnie saw three hands in an audience of 1,200 mental health clinicians, she said, wholly without sarcasm, "Wow — three! That's pretty good!" The audience burst out laughing in nervous camaraderie, but they knew it wasn't really funny.

The public is longing for new and better ways to *resolve* mental health challenges. For alternatives to conventional treatments. We frequently get asked questions about our findings. What all these people really need to know is: it is likely that many mental health problems might emerge *because our brains aren't getting the nutrients they need.*

• They won't often hear that from their mental health clinicians, because of a *second issue:* the persistent focus on life's stresses rather than how nutrition is the foundation of resilience. We hear all the time from people who want us to acknowledge that life is more complicated now: stress is everywhere, people are bullied and harassed, everyone is short of funds, and there is so much to worry about the future health of not just our bodies but of our planet. Our reaction? We tell them to think about their grandparents' generation who had the Great Depression, World Wars I and II, and the Holocaust to deal with. They didn't have many of the vaccines and antibiotics that we take for granted, since many of our most astonishing scientific discoveries and breakthroughs have come in recent decades. They didn't have computers or the internet for keeping in touch with family they left behind when they moved to North America.

Are our lives really more stressful than in previous generations? Or is our resilience lower due to our poor nutrient intake?

This book explains that optimal nutrition is fundamental for our brain cells to function well, so it just makes sense to focus on nutritional treatments. Even though they've been ignored or dismissed by many mental health clinicians, the data that have been published for years prove this. When emotional or mental health problems emerge, improve your nutrition *first*, before turning to medication. Optimizing nutrition is a safe and viable way to avoid, treat, or lessen mental illness. It is the magic ingredient for your resilience.

• *A third reason* nutrient treatments have not yet received the attention they deserve involves our system of health care. Pharmaceutical companies have a vested interest in patients being prescribed psychiatric medications. It earns them billions in profits, whereas they cannot make the same level of profit from most nutrient products, as we explain in chapters 1 and 11. And because psychiatrists have become primarily psychopharmacologists — trained in drug treatment in medical school and later by the pharmaceutical companies — it is understandable that they practice what they've been taught.

In general, the healthcare system in America operates within a model whereby psychiatric medications are typically prescribed after an initial diagnosis, followed by talk therapies and other support — if you're lucky and can afford to pay for it. Given that this approach is universal across all Western societies, however, you'd rightfully expect that it would be working well. In some cases, of course, these treatments do save lives and shouldn't be dismissed. But — and this is a *huge* but — if these treatments work really well, why are mental health problems increasing? Shouldn't they be decreasing instead?

From Hostility to Acceptance

At a national conference in December 2000, Bonnie presented a study of ten adults with bipolar disorder who got a lot better after they took one of the Alberta broad-spectrum multinutrient formulas. A reporter wrote up the findings in national Canadian news, and what happened next was not only astonishing but extremely painful — the media ridiculed Bonnie *and* the results. Worse, most Canadian psychiatrists told their patients *not* to take multinutrient formulas.

This hostility continued for years, even after Bonnie's rigorous studies were published in highly respected journals like the *Journal of Clinical Psychiatry* and *Journal of Child and Adolescent Psychopharmacology*, between 2001 and 2004.

The constant media coverage dismissing all the early studies meant that when a randomized placebo-controlled study began in 2004, not a single psychiatrist in Bonnie's city of over one million would refer patients. Even the bipolar disorder clinic in the city's largest teaching hospital told patients to stay away.

As mentioned, Julia began publishing about the effects of multinutrient formulas in 2009, and experienced some of the same attacks and hostility. In fact, one of the most consistent accusations has been that we work for the supplement companies. There is an amazing disbelief that we get no money from any of these companies.

Some of the reactions we continue to get when trying to present, publish, and fund our research have continued along these same lines. There is ridicule. There are ad hominem attacks. There are constant fears from others that we're going to harm people. And there are even accusations that we're *poisoning* people, which is ludicrously ironic considering how many people die after taking prescription meds every year! Just as ludicrous is that people flat-out tell us they don't believe the results of all our work, even though the numbers don't lie. That implies that we're falsifying data, one of the worst accusations that can be made against academic scientists.

Our heartbreaking experience with hostility is reminiscent of the German philosopher Schopenhauer's comment: All truth passes through three stages. First, it is ridiculed. Second, it is violently opposed. Third, it is accepted as being self-evident.

We hope this book moves everyone into the third stage.

Fortunately, this outmoded stance toward nutritional treatment is starting to change, though very slowly. Research appeared in 1992 showing that giving a few vitamins to patients on antidepressants resulted in them being able to *lower* their medications. Other studies done since then have validated the idea that giving people multiple nutrients enables them to *decrease their medications.*

If you are currently taking one or more psychiatric medications, this is a good-news story for you. Improving your diet and/or taking additional nutrients may allow you to lower your medication dose, or at least feel better at your current dose. In a PhD thesis supervised by Bonnie, Dr. Karen Davison, currently working at Kwantlen Polytechnic University in British Columbia, showed that in just three days, higher micronutrient intake was associated with better overall mental function in one hundred adults with mood disorders, most of whom were taking psychiatric meds. And we suspect that you feel a lot better when you eat well.

Of course you do. When your brain is well nourished, you need less medication.

Another major change has been that studies from many parts of the world are exploring combinations of nutrients for better brain health. In addition to studies of broad-spectrum formulas, there is also research on formulas with a smaller group of nutrients, especially the B-complex vitamins that we will tell you about in chapters 7 and 11.

As you will see in Part II, the shift in the last twenty years toward studying B-complex and broad-spectrum multinutrients has changed everything. That's because many researchers have finally realized that the "single ingredient solution" is no solution at all. Giving your brain *all* the nutrients it needs is what optimizes its health.

Both the public *and* our mental health experts need to learn that nutrition provides the foundation for brain health. This statement does not negate the importance of exercise, social support, meaningful work, and hobbies. But nutrition is fundamental for healthy cells. In fact, this book will show you that the impact of nutrition on brain function can be very rapid; the changes in mental health symptoms are sometimes almost immediate; and all of these benefits are proven by science — whether your doctors know that or not.

How to Use This Book

Part I, A Bold New Paradigm for Improving Mental Health, describes the basics of what nutrients do in your brain. Like almost all scientists, we also struggled with the concept of nutritional treatment of mental disorders when we first began our research, but once we engaged with the science, we realized that this kind of approach has amazing potential. We now know that some people may have underlying risk factors, perhaps genetic, that lead them to be more vulnerable to emotional distress when their diet is poor. Part I also discusses the importance of the microbiomes in your gut and in the soil, and how the gut and brain are surprisingly intertwined.

Part II, Better Nutrition for a Better Brain, presents many studies that have proven that nutrients really do make a difference in mental health. For example:

- In three randomized clinical trials of adults with depression and poor eating habits, education about how to improve their diet led to dramatic improvements in their mood in a matter of weeks. In many cases, complete remission of depression was achieved — they were no longer depressed at all.

- In one study on adults with ADHD, published in the *British Journal of Psychiatry* in April 2014, after only eight weeks, twice as many responded in the high-dose multinutrient group compared to the placebo group; twice as many went into remission in their depression; hyperactivity and impulsivity dropped into the normal range; and ADHD symptoms were less intrusive. Even better, at the one-year follow-up, those who stayed on micronutrients maintained their improvements or showed fewer symptoms compared to those who stopped or switched to medications and saw their symptoms get worse. They were also more likely to go into remission at follow-up on the nutrients. And these short- and long-term findings have recently been replicated in a study conducted with children with ADHD.

- In two studies, one with 358 adults with bipolar symptoms and the second with 120 children with bipolar symptoms, micronutrients reduced symptoms on average by 50 percent, and this was sustained for six months with a simultaneous reduction in the use of medications.

- Nutrients given to survivors after natural disasters or traumatic events are proof that a well-nourished body and brain are better able to recover from major stress events. Even after a year, people who received the nutrients did better than those who didn't.

- Every clinical trial using *broad-spectrum* multinutrients to treat people who have psychiatric symptoms has shown positive results. The research has reported that approximately 80 percent of people experience some benefit from treatment, with about 50 percent being much to very much improved when taking the multinutrient formulas. That's how powerful this treatment is.

In Part III, How to Feed Your Brain, you'll learn why it's time to stop putting the whole world on pills. Looking at *any* class of psychiatric drugs, whether they're antidepressants, antipsychotics, or anti-anxiety medications, the pattern is the same. In the short term, these drugs are often very effective, with some people experiencing dramatic improvement in their psychiatric symptoms. But in the long term, too often, they aren't. And in some cases, they make life much worse for those who take them.

Although medications may help reduce many symptoms, they often don't restore people to normal mental health. There must be a better way. And there is. Instead of pharmaceuticals, good nutrition is an *essential* part of recovery and continued healthy brain function.

You don't need us to tell you about the typical Western diet. You already know that it's high in calories, refined grains, and sugar; it's heavily processed; and it's low in fresh produce, especially vegetables. In contrast, a healthy, Mediterranean-style diet is high in fresh vegetables and fruits, nuts, good fats, and fish. It's low in ultra-processed foods and sugary drinks. And here is the scary fact — government data from the United States, Canada, New Zealand, and Australia show that *at least* 50 percent of what we now put into our mouths *does not even qualify as food*. It is ultra-processed "stuff." Stuff made from simple carbs (sugar), salt, trans fats, and chemicals like artificial coloring.

Food is defined as nutritious substances we consume for growth and to maintain life. There has not been a single study showing that the Western diet is good for our mental health. Those who eat a Mediterranean diet, on the other hand, have lower rates of depression than those who eat Western diets.

Our food supply is also a factor in our decreased nutrient intake. Climate change, increasing levels of carbon dioxide in the atmosphere, and poor soil quality lower the nutrient density of what we eat, which means that the apple you eat today doesn't have the same nutrients as one eaten a generation or two ago. So we need to improve our soil, in order to grow and eat healthier food.

These chapters will show you how to rethink your food choices, give your pantry the makeover it needs, and make shopping and cooking a breeze. The food plans and recipes make this even easier — and delicious.

In Part III we will also tell you about the supplements that have been studied, whether you need to do blood testing beforehand, and any side effects you need to be concerned about if you decide to use supplements.

We want this book to be the tipping point for revolutionizing the way mental health problems are treated. Not only will this book show you how to take prevention seriously by optimizing your nutrient intake, but it will give you the information you need so that you can have informed discussions with all your healthcare providers about options that might really work for you.

This book will put the critical knowledge in *your* hands, and it will empower you to improve not only your life but the lives of your loved ones.

Making this happen is why we wrote this book. To work toward a more successful treatment approach, one that is more affordable and accessible to the millions of people who need it.

When people realize what nutrients do inside their brains, they are more likely to change the way they eat. People get better not just in terms of mental health symptoms — their sleep improves; their moods improve; their need for addictive drugs like cigarettes, marijuana, and alcohol goes down; and they find it much easier to cope with life's daily stresses.

We can do better if we learn how to care for our brains through nutrition. Change is long overdue. And no prescription is needed!

Part I

A BOLD NEW PARADIGM FOR IMPROVING MENTAL HEALTH

1

THE MISSING KEY FOR MENTAL HEALTH

> What is probably inherited in mental illness are genes that regulate
> brain metabolism of essential nutrients.
>
> — NOBEL PRIZE WINNER DR. LINUS PAULING, 1968

IF WE HAD A dollar for every time a psychiatrist has said to us: "Those vitamins and minerals you're studying — they can't actually affect the brain, can they?" we'd be able to fund a great deal of research!

Many people find it hard to believe that "*just*" nutrition could solve mental health problems. This attitude isn't just wrong. It's *wrong, outdated, and harmful* — especially because there have been dozens and dozens of rigorous scientific studies showing that nutrition can be a vital key for preventing and treating mental disorders.

But we know why these psychiatrists think this way.

Like them, we're products of that same type of education. While in graduate school, we were barely taught about nutrition. And the few hours that were spent on it taught us that nutrition was not relevant for mental health, and that psychiatric symptoms were manifestations of chemical imbalances in the brain that could only be corrected with medications. Physicians are no different from the rest of us: for everyone, our knowledge is heavily influenced by the courses we took in school. For the last fifty years, much of that curriculum for physicians, as well as their continuing medical education, has been sponsored by pharmaceutical companies. What does this mean? It means that what they're taught is that the treatment for brain health must focus on drugs.

It's frustrating that physicians are usually not taught the very basics of nutrition. In the 2014 call to action entitled "A Deficiency of Nutrition Education in Medical Training" published in the *American Journal of Medicine,* multiple studies were summarized showing that nutrition was the single most important factor in disability and premature death, and could explain well over half of the cases of cardiovascular disease.[1] In spite of this powerful information relating diet to physical health, medical schools were devoting fewer than twenty hours of their four-year training to nutrition. *And what about mental health?* Our brains demand a disproportionately large amount of the nutrients we consume, so the need for nutrition education related to *mental* health is even greater.

The lack of nutrition education isn't limited to psychiatrists and family physicians. Other mental health professionals usually don't learn about nutrition either. Teachers don't learn about it — so their students don't learn about it in school. As a result, most Americans don't know that the brain metabolism responsible for the production of neurotransmitters like serotonin and dopamine is dependent on an ample supply of micronutrients (which you will learn about in chapter 2).

Like almost all scientists, we both struggled with the concept of nutritional treatment when we first began our research. Once we engaged with the science, however, its potential was undeniably clear. We now know that there are many people with underlying risk factors, often genetic, that may make them more vulnerable to emotional distress when their diet is poor. Improve and fix their nutritional needs, and many of them can and will get better.

First the Bad News: The Tsunami of Mental Disorders Has Hit

Despite billions of research dollars over the years, we still don't know what precisely causes mental illness. Science has uncovered some clues, like our genetics, our childhood environment, exposure to traumas, poverty, social deprivation, and the effects of toxins on neural development. And the numbers appear to be rising.

Some of the most sobering data on the prevalence of mental disorders come from a book by Dr. E. Fuller Torrey and Judy Miller published in 2001. They collected government data from all over the world and found consistent evidence for a mental illness prevalence rate of 1 in 10,000 up to the year 1750 — but that rate tripled from 1 to 3 in 10,000 between 1750 and 1960. This increase worried them so much that they entitled their book *The Invisible Plague.*

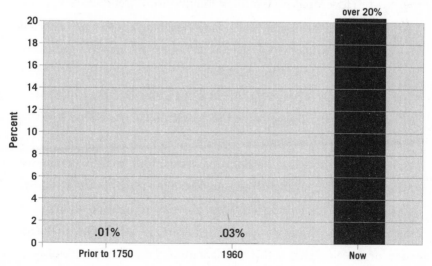

Prevalence of Diagnosed Mental Illness

What about now? Actually, 3 in 10,000 sounds wonderful in comparison with the latest World Health Organization report of over *2,000 in every 10,000*. That's a shocking one in five, or 20 percent of us! If you look at the lifetime occurrence, the CDC says it is 5,000 in every 10,000. Yes, *50 percent*.

If our current treatments are really effective, why isn't the rate of mental disorders going down? Why has the diagnosis of mental health conditions increased so dramatically in the last sixty years?

All of this means that the rates of people on disability as a direct consequence of a mental disorder are on the rise. Insurance costs are on the rise. Treatment costs are catastrophic.

The plague is no longer invisible, and it is continuing to get worse. This really is a tsunami. Although some of the increase is certainly due to our more open society, more mental health professionals diagnosing disorders, and a willingness of people to seek help — which is a really good thing, of course — such staggering numbers suggest that other things are going on. Like how and what we eat.

How Mental Health Problems Are Categorized

Why do you need to know how mental health symptoms are classified? Because health insurance companies will not reimburse for medical appointments without a diagnostic label.

The diagnostic reference for medical practitioners in the United States is the DSM, or the *Diagnostic and Statistical Manual of Mental Disorders*, currently in its fifth edition.

The DSM presents a classification system, prepared by committees who try to come up with a consensus. The increase in the diagnostic categories from the first edition in 1952 until the most current edition in 2013 is startling: the number has quadrupled from 128 to 541. One of the reasons for these updates is that the definition of a mental health disorder reflects the times and the culture. For instance, homosexuality was classified as a psychiatric disorder from 1968 until it was removed in 1987. Did homosexuality change? No, our culture did. Also, some new categories have been added, recognizing that meds can cause adverse side effects.

The most familiar categories are:

- Anxiety disorders, including panic disorder, obsessive-compulsive disorder, post-traumatic stress disorder, and phobias
- Depression, bipolar disorder, and other mood disorders
- Eating disorders
- Personality disorders like narcissistic and antisocial personality disorders
- Psychotic disorders, including schizophrenia
- Neurodevelopmental disorders like ADHD and autism spectrum disorder (ASD)
- Medication-induced movement disorders, and other adverse effects of medications

Why Our Current Approach Isn't Working

Julia's TEDx talk was about her research establishing that many of the people given extra minerals and vitamins showed a reduction in their mental symptoms. Since the talk went public at the end of 2014, she has received thousands of phone calls, emails, and messages on Facebook, Instagram, and Twitter telling her detailed, painful, and deeply personal stories, and asking for advice. They tell of lives being devastated by mental illness and the ensuing treatments. They tell of trying to cope with multiple medications that create increasingly problematic side effects, like weight gain and diabetes, and how they're then given *more* medications to address the side effects of the other meds. They tell of the years wasted because treatments didn't give them the quality of life that all of us aspire to. They tell of becoming a shell of who they were and getting further and further away from their full potential.

Most heartbreaking is that they tell of hopelessness.

Julia is also a practicing clinical psychologist, and she has seen that psychiatric medications can help some people tremendously, saving their lives. But in twenty-five years as a practicing clinician, this happens less frequently than we would hope.

When she was recently a collaborator on a study looking at whether genetics or personality could predict who would develop side effects to antidepressants (they didn't), Julia was dismayed by one of the most telling points. About two hundred people were in the study; 70.8 percent of them fell above the "high psychological distress" range, with half of these people falling in the "very high distress" range (indicative of a severe mental disorder).[2] But most of them (84.5 percent) were already taking antidepressants — the typical, conventional treatment — so the medications clearly were not resolving their mood problems!

Why has our society not noticed that our current conventional approaches don't lead to recovery? If these drugs were conventional treatments for an infection yet the infections continued, people would be demanding something better. But when it comes to mental disorders, we seem to accept that partial or minimal recovery is adequate. Well, it isn't.

How Conventional Treatment Failed a
Little Boy—but Nutrients Didn't

Andrew was a ten-year-old boy who suffered from anxiety and symptoms of psychosis, coupled with frequent intrusive thoughts and compulsions typical of OCD (obsessive-compulsive disorder). He had spent six months in a children's hospital, with no improvement whatsoever, when his mother, who'd heard about micronutrient treatment, telephoned Bonnie in desperation.

She was not just desperate to find a treatment that would help her child; she was desperate for an expert to validate the use of these nutrients. They had an appointment scheduled with Dr. Megan Rodway, a child and adolescent psychiatrist, but were afraid that she would refuse to help them if they wanted their son treated with nutrients. Thankfully, Dr. Rodway, although highly skeptical of the efficacy of the multinutrient formula (she called it "snake oil"), had the integrity to acknowledge that medications had not helped Andrew . . . so why not try the nutrients?

Improvements in Andrew's mental health began very quickly after starting the broad-spectrum multinutrient formula. Within ten months, his OCD symptoms had virtually disappeared. Over about eleven months, so did his symptoms of psychosis.

What six months of inpatient treatment couldn't resolve, minerals and vitamins were able to fix. Not only that, but the nutrient treatment cost less than 2 percent of his inpatient treatment.[3]

A decade later, Andrew still takes his nutrients, and when he does, he has no symptoms of psychosis — meaning that he is able to function in the real world — although he is still challenged by anxiety. He graduated from high school (which is very rare for someone with childhood psychosis), works part-time, volunteers at his church, and has friends.

Yet, even after Andrew improved so drastically, and everyone in the psychiatry department at the hospital knew this, they did not change their mental health treatment practices. (Read about what happened to Dr. Rodway in chapter 12.) In fact, Bonnie asked a young psychiatrist at that hospital if he would then consider using nutrients with any other cases, knowing how well they worked for Andrew. His response was no, not until nutritional treatment was in the clinical practice guidelines (CPGs). This is unlikely to happen anytime soon, because it all boils down to money (more about this in the section "One Way Money Influences Diagnosis and Treatment" later in this chapter). And his comment revealed a disheartening double standard, as psychiatrists often go outside the CPGs, such as using meds for children that have been approved only in adults or using meds "off label," which means prescribing them for an illness that has insufficient science to support this prescribing.

Good Nutrition = Good Brain Health
Has Been Known for Centuries!

That nutrition is relevant to health is not a new idea. The father of modern medicine, Hippocrates (c. 460–c. 370 BCE), knew what he was talking about when he said, "Let food be thy medicine and medicine thy food." Although we'll never know whether he considered *mental* health, he certainly had the right attitude about nutrition.

Our more immediate ancestors have known for many centuries that nutrition was a big part of the mental health picture. During medieval times, for instance, physicians stressed climate and exercise, alongside diet and herbal medicines, for the promotion of health and for the treatment of disorders.[4] In the nineteenth century and into the early twentieth century, the conventional wisdom was that mental symptoms were manifestations of inadequate nutrition.[5]

In fact, the fastest way for us to help people (and to eliminate the stigma of mental illness!) would be to return to the diagnosis described in *The People's Home Library* over a hundred years ago in North America: people with mental health symptoms were told they were suffering from "imperfect nutrition" and they should eat a better diet.

What happened in the mid-twentieth century? Taking prescription medications for all sorts of conditions became much more common and socially acceptable. It also marked the beginning of drug development targeting the brain.

As a result of this new-drug explosion, the use of nutrients and good nutrition as a treatment disappeared from common knowledge. Since, as you've learned already, medical students were barely given a cursory lecture on nutrition in their four years of study, they had no idea nutrients were even an option. Instead, pharmaceutical companies began to control the narrative by providing the funding for much of the continuing medical education of our physicians.[6]

Also relevant is the fact that most nutrient products cannot be patented. Suppose your company makes a natural nutrient product containing 100 mg of vitamin C, and you go through the lengthy and expensive process of patenting your formula. All that a second manufacturer would have to do to produce a virtually identical product (without being guilty of violating your patent) would be to include a slight variation of the content, perhaps 105 mg of vitamin C. In other words, with most natural products, patent "protection" and the anticipated profits provide no protection at all.

Think about this: How is it possible that every product from pharmaceutical companies has been assumed to represent good science, while anything about nutrition is assumed to be a scam? What has gone wrong with our scientists and our medical societies that these attitudes have prevailed?

If you've ever gotten a prescription for a medication that didn't work, or if you had side effects that were worse than the initial illness or injury, you might have already asked yourself these questions. One of the reasons our Western society and so many of our physicians are often hostile toward nutrient-based treatments for mental health symptoms is that they don't fit with their education or their worldview. In addition, people who find that a better diet and supplements have improved their mental health are often able to stop taking medications, so proving the effectiveness of a nutritional approach has the capacity to hit the pharmaceutical industry in their pocketbooks.

The "Single Ingredient Solution" Is No Solution at All

Physicians and scientists in the modern era tend to think in terms of single ingredient solutions — in other words, a magic bullet. You have an infection? Take an antibiotic. You have postoperative pain? Take a painkiller. You have angina? Put a nitroglycerin tablet under your tongue. Worried about birth defects? Take folic acid.

It is hard to overestimate how much this magic bullet thinking has contributed to burying knowledge about nutrition and mental health. It's profound — and for all the wrong reasons.

Bonnie's review of the treatment studies for mental disorders from 1920 to 2000 found hundreds of publications reporting studies of one nutrient at a time, such as calcium, manganese, iron, zinc, magnesium, etc.[7] Sometimes there were a few modest improvements, but not enough to change clinical practice.

Why was so much time and effort dedicated to studying one nutrient at a time? The single-nutrient mindset was formed in part by the discovery of dramatic cures for single-nutrient deficiency diseases: scurvy is 100 percent preventable with enough vitamin C, for instance, and pellagra is 100 percent eliminated with enough vitamin B3 (niacin).

But we know now that no *single* nutrient can successfully treat the complexity of brain and mental disorders. Studying them individually, one by one, was exactly the *wrong* way to go about it — because there is no single magic bullet solution. As you'll see in the next chapter, nutrients work together synergistically. They need each other to function. This is why we're not reviewing all the single-nutrient clinical trials; we now know the results are rarely as helpful as those done on combinations of multiple nutrients.

The magic bullet approach has never made sense in terms of how the brain works. It also doesn't make sense in terms of how we eat. If you're deficient in one nutrient, it is almost certain that you're also going to be deficient in many other nutrients because they are closely correlated in our diets.

One Way Money Influences Diagnosis and Treatment

Consumers should know that the clinical practice guidelines (CPGs) referred to above are usually written by committees — often with financial ties to pharmaceutical companies.

Psychiatrist Allen Frances, the author of *Saving Normal: An Insider's Revolt Against Out-of-Control Psychiatric Diagnosis, DSM-5, Big Pharma, and the Medicalization of Ordinary Life,* published in 2014, said that 56 percent of the experts working on the task force he led to update the DSM had financial ties to drug companies. On June 20, 2017, an article entitled "The Pressure of Big Pharma," published in the Canadian national newspaper the *Globe and Mail,* reported that 59 percent of the twenty-two CPG members who developed the mental health treatment guidelines in Canada received funding from pharmaceutical companies.

That number doesn't begin to tell the whole story. Of the remaining nine who declared no financial conflicts, seven were psychologists; in other words, people who cannot even legally prescribe medication in Canada, so they aren't a target of pharmaceutical funding. So in reality, only two of the twenty-two panelists had rejected pharmaceutical money. Most panelists had ties to many different companies; one, in fact, had ties to *seventeen* of them!

What chance is there that currently constituted CPG committees, funded heavily by pharmaceutical companies, will ever include nutrient treatment in their CPGs, no matter how strong the evidence? We know the answer. Even though there are enough controlled trials right now to meet FDA requirements for proving efficacy, those results have had little impact on CPGs. Money talks.

The Alliance of Psychopharmacologists and
Direct-to-Consumer Advertising

One of the obstacles to improving mental health treatment is that psychiatrists in this century are primarily psychopharmacologists, trained in drug treatment when they are in medical school and later by the pharmaceutical companies that make the medications. Direct-to-consumer (DTC) advertising, approved in the United States in 1985 and escalating in 1997 when the FDA removed some restrictions, resulted in the saturation of the public with ads touting the wonders of the latest and greatest medications.

This combination of psychiatrists as psychopharmacologists along with a public bombarded by ads for new "miracle" drugs has influenced many people to think that they really *must* try the latest new medications to solve their problems.

The saturation of our media by drug advertising has also influenced people's reactions to nutrition research — they can't believe something so simple might solve their enormous problems. We have witnessed the fury of some whose mood disorder symptoms were finally controlled by nutrients — fury, in particular, at their prescribing physicians, who never told them about the role of nutrition in brain function.

Believing that nutrition is a useless treatment for mental health stems from this:

First, the DTC marketing has convinced consumers that if they have a psychiatric problem, they need meds, and that wonder drugs exist for every mental problem.

Second, DTC advertising has also led to disease-mongering, which has been a great marketing success and has resulted in exponential increases in the public demand for meds.

Third, many medical professionals still adhere to the erroneous belief that if you eat a balanced diet, you don't need any supplements. And that if you do take them, they're going to hurt or even kill you. (More about this in chapter 11).

Fourth, as you've learned already, there is a lack of education in medical schools about the vital need for good nutrition for brain health.

Bottom line: Those suffering from years of mental problems think that nutrients are too trivial to be useful for their problems. So do their doctors. Read on, and you will see why this simply isn't true.

How Well Do Psych Meds Really Work? Or Do They?

For the past fifty years, announcements of new psychiatric medications have often been greeted as the new miracle cure. Only in the past few years has the pendulum begun to swing in the other direction, with both scientists and the public recognizing that they haven't turned out to be as good as we hoped they would be. In spite of the fact that many people benefit from psychiatric meds, especially during short-term crises, in group studies the difference in impact between antidepressants and a placebo is usually a few points on a depression rating scale: statistically significant, but clinically trivial.

It might also shock you to learn that most psychiatric medications are approved by the FDA based on clinical trials that lasted a mere six to twelve weeks — but psychiatrists may tell their patients to take the medications *for life!* Psychiatrists, after all, want their patients to feel better and stay better.

We often think of antipsychotic medications as a life-saving treatment for people suffering from schizophrenia (and we sometimes judge people harshly if things go wrong and it's assumed that they "went off their meds"). But even these treatments are not as effective as we hope. For example, with schizophrenia, antipsychotics can reduce hallucinations and delusions within weeks, but around 80 percent of patients show a relapse in these symptoms within the first few years of treatment.[8] (Contrast that result with Andrew, who still has complete control of hallucinations and delusions with nutrients, even after more than ten years.)

But there are many sides to this story.

First, there is no doubt that many people in crisis benefit from short-term administration of a sedative, or something to help with sleep. This is usually called "acute" treatment, meant for a short time only, with the intention to wean the patient off the meds.

Second, some people benefit from psychiatric medications over time, with no side effects. These people are a minority, but for them, conventional medications are a good option.

The Potential for Harm

What if some of the psychiatric medications that are prescribed actually make people *worse*?

A number of researchers, especially in Europe, have questioned both the short-term and the long-term use of meds, highlighting some of the significant harm that they can cause, including increased aggression and suicidality in adults.[9] People taking antidepressants have a higher suicide rate than those who do not, especially in the first month of medication use, and even in studies where they don't know if they're taking meds or a placebo.[10] A more recent re-analysis of FDA data showed that the rate of attempted suicide was about 2.5 times higher with antidepressant use relative to placebo.[11] There have also been many incidents reported in the media of parents killing/harming their children or children killing/harming their parents while in a psychotic state due to prescribed psychiatric meds.[12]

Psychiatric meds can also cause severe metabolic side effects, leading to rapid weight gain. In addition, one of the most significant problems of these drugs is constipation. This can kill patients — and it does[13] — leading to recommendations that people prescribed an antipsychotic should take a laxative alongside their antipsychotic prescription.

Meds can also lead to a host of new problems. Professor John Read and his colleagues have published surveys of large groups of children and adults taking psychiatric medications, and the results are astonishing in terms of the high proportion of individuals reporting suicidal thinking (39 percent), feeling emotionally numb (60 percent), caring less about others (39 percent), loss of libido (62 percent), and so on.[14]

Governments also have been signaling lately that medications have not had the effect that we all hoped they would have. A 2018 report to the New Zealand government stated: "We can't medicate . . . our way out of the epidemic of mental distress."[15]

The distinction between short- and long-term use of psychiatric meds is increasingly important. Studies such as one in the Netherlands showed that seven years after a first episode of psychosis, people who had been randomly assigned to a treatment plan where their meds were gradually decreased or completely removed were more likely to get a job or return to school, and generally did better in society, than those who were maintained on their full dose of psychiatric meds.[16] In other words, acute use may make sense, but for some people, long-term exposure to psychiatric medications can be an impediment to living a full and productive life.

Dr. Frances, the author of *Saving Normal*, said in 2013, "There has been no real advance in diagnosis since DSM-III in 1980, and no real advance in treatment since the early 1990s." This comment is a scathing indictment of psychiatric medication, made by a very knowledgeable individual, although it is pretty clear that he is not familiar with the research on nutrient treatment.

Why Is It So Hard to Get Off Psychiatric Medications?

Anyone prescribed psychiatric meds is sternly warned never to go off them cold turkey, as there could be dire side effects.

Yet when Bonnie was researching withdrawal symptoms twenty years ago, she couldn't find any information. At all. Literally not one single reference in the medical literature about any withdrawal effects, even though it was common knowledge passed along from physicians to patients. How was this possible?

In a chance encounter with a psychiatrist colleague, she asked him about it and was told she had to use the proper search term: "discontinuation syndrome." Not *withdrawal*.

This was completely ludicrous, because every other addictive substance was identified as having withdrawal symptoms, but somehow the entire medical community had been convinced to avoid the term "withdrawal" when the drug in question was for mental health.

Discontinuation syndrome is a deceptive way to classify the seriousness of withdrawal. Scientific research now shows that more than half (56 percent) of people who try to come off antidepressants have withdrawal effects, and nearly half (46 percent) of those who do have withdrawal effects describe them as severe.[17] A *Psychology Today* article published on August 26, 2019, described the hostility from the field of psychiatry when confronted with the data on antidepressant withdrawal (AW) as follows:

> This is what happens when a preferred narrative collapses under the weight of long-suppressed counter-evidence. Those who have invested decades and careers in its assumptions are likely to try to cling to its illusions, seemingly unaware that in doing so they're misinforming their patients on the high probability of AW and other adverse effects.

There is now a whole field of de-prescribing (safe medication tapers) for psychiatrists to study.[18] It's great that physicians now recognize that withdrawal symptoms are real, but there's only been minimal interest about using or even researching whether nutrients can ease withdrawal symptoms.

We're not surprised. They are not considering the use of nutrients for withdrawal possibly for the same reasons they don't use them in the first place: nutrition is simply not taught sufficiently in medical schools.[19] But this is an area that ought to be explored, as there are some hints about reduced cravings in well-nourished people. Anecdotally, people tell us they've been able to cut back on cigarettes, cannabis, and alcohol when taking multinutrient supplements, suggesting there may be a role for nutrients in helping with drug withdrawal symptoms. (For more, see chapter 6.)

Now the Good News: Many Mental Health Problems Can Be Prevented or Treated

Read on, and we'll show you how eating better food and supplementing with micronutrients can help your mental health. But it has been a long road to get even this far . . .

There have been many reports in the United States over the last five to ten years on the state of our physical health. How and what people eat is *the* most significant risk factor for premature death and disability. Usually, these reports have focused on cardiovascular problems because that's where there's a huge amount of information linking food and health. A 2013 report on the state of US health identified dietary factors as the single most significant risk factor for disability and premature death.[20]

Here's what you're *not* told. How and what you eat is also an important risk factor for *mental* disorders. But this is actually good news *because you can do something about it!*

Knowledge is truly power. All of us can reduce our risk of cardiovascular disease once we're armed with the information we need to change our diets, increase our exercise, and enhance our social networks. You can do the exact same thing for the health of your brain.

You can easily change how and what you eat. You can change other lifestyle factors too, like the amount of exercise and sleep you get, and the things you can do to minimize stress. These factors are *modifiable. We* can't change the way *you* eat. But we can give you the knowledge that will help you understand:

- The importance of improving your brain health
- What nutrients do for your brain every minute that you are alive
- What nutrients do to modify the expression of your inherited genes
- How nutrients improve your resilience
- What nutrients do to help protect you from toxins
- Which nutrients you should be looking for in your diet
  . . . and much more.

The Takeaway

1. Mental health diagnoses are on the rise, and current conventional medical treatments aren't working sufficiently well to actually resolve the problem for many. With at least 20 percent of Americans currently struggling with a mental health challenge, it's probably a conservative estimate that more than 50 percent of the population is suffering, because when one person is challenged, a whole family feels the impact.

2. Money influences how mental challenges are diagnosed and treated. Even though there is overwhelming evidence that psychiatric medications aren't always very effective, can have serious effects, and haven't been rigorously tested over long periods of time, this knowledge has not translated into a change in prescribing practices. Clinical practice guidelines, which define how clinicians should treat mental health

problems, are heavily influenced by individuals receiving funds from pharmaceutical companies.

3. That food can effectively treat mental health issues has been known for *centuries,* so it's time for mainstream medicine to stop ignoring this basic information. Nutrition still isn't a critical component of curricula for people studying to be physicians or psychologists. Another obstacle is that both scientists and clinicians keep searching for a single magic bullet—one nutrient that will resolve a mental health problem. Humans are inclined to look for simple solutions, but the brain is much more complex.

4. Fortunately, once you feed your brain what it needs, you can treat and even prevent many different mental health problems. After you read this book, the power to improve your mental health will be in your own hands.

2

FOOD FOR THOUGHT: THE NUTRIENTS YOUR BRAIN NEEDS

There is not a single controlled study showing that stress *causes* any form of insanity, although . . . stress can make the illness worse.

— E. FULLER TORREY AND JUDY MILLER, *The Invisible Plague*

BY NOW, YOU HAVE probably read lots of articles about people eating better and feeling better physically. You probably noticed that a general rule is to avoid heavily processed, packaged foods (sometimes referred to as junk food), and to concentrate instead on real, whole foods. We all accept that eating this type of a healthy diet is important for our cardiovascular system, our muscles, our bones. But have you ever thought about your *brain* health in this way?

Do you know the basic science behind what your brain needs for it to work at its very best? If you don't, you're not alone. This information needs to be taught in elementary schools, in high schools, and certainly in medical schools — but it rarely is. After you know what nutrients actually do in your brain, we're pretty sure you'll feel motivated to seek them out.

The most important thing to know is this: we need the full spectrum of minerals and vitamins every minute of every day to fully optimize our brain function, especially under stress.

So let's begin with some building blocks.

Your Hungry Brain

Every minute of your life, your bloodstream distributes oxygen and nutrients to every part of your brain and body. Think of your brain as an insatiable glutton — but not in a bad way, because the more you feed it with the nutrients it needs, the better it will serve you.

Brain development requires many, many nutrients, and essential fatty acids in particular. Essential fatty acids (EFAs), omega-3, and omega-6 are all terms that refer to a group of compounds especially critical for building cell membranes and ensuring the proper function of these membranes. Humans can't synthesize omega-3 fatty acids, which means the only way we can get them is through food or supplementation.

These fatty acids play an especially important role in the central nervous system, particularly in building the brains of fetuses and young children. And it may surprise you to learn that critical aspects of brain development, especially in our frontal lobes, continue until we are in our late twenties. Even after that age, essential fatty acids do not lose their importance for brain function.

As recently as a decade ago, most people were unfamiliar with the term "omega-3s," but now you're more likely to know, at least, that they're something that's good for you.

Just as important is knowing that your body needs an optimal balance between omega-3 and omega-6 fatty acids. For mental health, there are two omega-3 fatty acids, DHA (docosahexaenoic acid) and EPA (eicosapentaenoic acid), that are especially important.

Ample data have shown that, ideally, the balance in our diets should be 1:1, or perhaps 2:1, of omega-6 to omega-3. But a Western diet that is very high in processed food and very low in fish usually has an omega-6 to omega-3 ratio that is around 15:1 or even higher. In other words, the more processed food you eat, the more likely you are to be consuming excessive amounts of omega-6 fatty acids. This is an incredibly worrying statistic, as these high ratios of omega-6 to omega-3 have been associated with cardiovascular disease, excessive inflammation, and many forms of cancer.[1]

Before we continue telling you all the amazing things nutrients do for your brain, we need to define "nutrient." Given that most dietary advice focuses on carbohydrates, proteins, and fats, many people might think these are the nutrients we need to make sure we eat. But that is only half of the story.

Carbs, proteins, and fats are *macro*nutrients. Macro means large, for large molecules. And yes, they are essential for your brain to develop and operate. Carbs provide glucose; proteins give us amino acids; and fats are required for overall brain structure, among many other functions.

The almost exclusive focus on these three macronutrients is at the expense of much smaller but essential nutrients, or *micro*nutrients. Minerals and vitamins are sometimes called micronutrients, because we often require them in much smaller quantities; you may have heard the term "trace minerals" for some, indicating those are needed in really tiny amounts.

The difference between vitamins and minerals gets into some biochemical terms:

- Vitamins are organic molecules (meaning they contain carbon) and are very susceptible to heat — overcooking breaks them down.
- In contrast, minerals are stable chemical elements you might remember from the periodic table that was probably on the wall in your high school chemistry class. They do not break down as easily as vitamins do. As you will learn in chapter 3, plants absorb the minerals they find in the soil and use them to produce vitamins. Hu-

mans cannot do that, although if we have a healthy digestive system, some of those little organisms in our gut (more on this in chapter 3) manufacture small amounts of vitamins for us. But we need to keep in mind that plants are the original food manufacturer for humans, long before we had McDonald's!

Where this gets confusing is that ultra-processed foods do contain carbs, proteins, and fats, but many lack essential *micronutrients*. Adding to this confusion is that some minerals are considered to be macrominerals (e.g., calcium, phosphorus, magnesium, potassium) since they are bulkier than the trace minerals (like zinc, copper, iodine, and selenium). But we will consistently refer to minerals and vitamins as micronutrients.

Vitamins are organic compounds that we humans need every day for optimal growth and development, and that we mainly cannot synthesize ourselves. This means we have to eat them. Most are water soluble, so that if we consume more than we need we simply excrete the excess. A few, like vitamin A and vitamin D, are fat (or lipid) soluble, meaning that an excess will be stored in our fat cells. (That is why those who consume enormously excessive and never-recommended amounts of fat-soluble vitamins over the years can put themselves at risk for an overdose.)

B vitamins are tricky to understand because there are so many of them, and some are best known as a number, like vitamin B12, while others are best known by their name, such as thiamine (which is actually vitamin B1) — even though most B vitamins have both a name and a number. These are the most common B vitamins:

- Vitamin B1 (thiamine)
- Vitamin B2 (riboflavin)
- Vitamin B3 (niacin)
- Vitamin B5 (pantothenic acid)
- Vitamin B6 (pyridoxine)

- Vitamin B7 (biotin)
- Vitamin B9 (folate, or folic acid, which is the synthetic form)
- Vitamin B12 (cyanocobalamin)

In addition, there are other compounds referred to as "vitamin-like" because they haven't been categorized as vitamins yet, but scientists seem to think that's how they function. Examples are choline, inositol, and co-enzyme Q10.

Why You Need to Feed Your Brain

Because it is so important to understand that we eat to feed our brains, let's take a look at five of the critical ways in which *micro*nutrients make our brains healthy.

Enabling Your Brain to Function

Throughout brain development and until the end of your life, a *quart* of blood passes through your brain every single minute that your heart is beating. That quart represents 15 to 20 percent of all the blood inside you, but your brain is only about 2 percent of your body weight. Believe it or not, your brain is actually a very small organ! What we sometimes say is that our brains "punch above their weight," needing to be fed as much as ten times the amount of blood you would expect for an organ so small. And even though it is so small, if all its blood vessels were laid out flat they would stretch about four hundred miles.

Here's the important question: Why have we evolved to require such an enormous amount of blood to bathe our brains every minute of our lives? That quart of blood is bringing the nutrients and oxygen to every single nook and cranny in your cranium. Now ask yourself: What have you eaten in the last day or so? *That* is what you are feeding your brain!

As the most metabolically active organ in your body, your brain is constantly and disproportionately demanding oxygen and nutrients. In fact, this little organ uses 20 to 40 percent of the nutrients and energy you consume — and remember, it is only about 2 percent of your body weight. So this is the key message: even though we do need to eat properly to build a strong musculoskeletal system and a healthy cardiovascular system, *when we eat, we are primarily feeding our brains.* And that is very important, because our brain plays a major role in how we see, smell, hear, taste, think, feel, learn, remember, process, and create.

Brain function is dependent on *brain metabolism.*

Metabolism is merely the *transformation* of one compound to another. In every organ of our body, including our brain, chemicals go through multiple conversions. Perhaps the one you are most familiar with involves the amino acid called tryptophan. Tryptophan is converted into a neurotransmitter, the chemical messenger between brain cells, called serotonin. We do not eat serotonin directly; our very clever bodies are chemical laboratories that can take the chemicals that we consume, like tryptophan, and convert them into other chemicals like the neurotransmitters. I'm glad "I" don't have to do it — I wouldn't know how!

To convert tryptophan into serotonin, there has to be a catalyst for this reaction to take place. Enter the enzymes. Their role is to do the conversion work. But enzymes cannot do their job without a steady supply of cofactors — which are micronutrients (minerals and vitamins).

In other words: *you need to feed your brain a steady supply of micronutrients to provide the cofactors needed for optimal brain metabolism.*

Think about it like fuel for your car: you can have the best car in the world but it won't run if it's out of gas. It's that simple.

Only with the proper nutrients do you have a chance of providing your brain with the building blocks it requires for good functioning. And since our bodies don't make minerals at all and they make very few vitamins, we *must* get these micronutrients from our *food.*

Let's use serotonin to help explain this process in more detail. This is a particularly good example, because serotonin is a well-known neurotransmitter that plays a significant role in mood. SSRIs, or selective *serotonin reuptake inhibitors*, are a category of psychiatric medication. An SSRI is supposed to increase the availability of serotonin in the spaces (synapses) between brain cells (neurons), by blocking the reabsorption and metabolism of the serotonin that's there.

But what if instead of blocking the breakdown of serotonin to keep more of it available to neurons, you increased its availability by manufacturing more of it by increasing your nutrient intake? Remember, minerals and vitamins are the cofactors that enable your brain to manufacture more serotonin and other chemicals. So improving your diet likely influences your supply of serotonin.[2]

The figure on the next page is a simplified diagram of how tryptophan is converted to serotonin, and how they are both then broken down into other by-products. Although we don't list the enzymes because the figure would get too complicated, think of every arrow as representing a metabolic step controlled by enzymes. The nutrients that are the cofactors for those enzymes are in dashed-line boxes. The figure shows you how the minerals and vitamins from your food all work together in metabolic pathways.

To convert tryptophan to serotonin, you need three minerals (iron, phosphorus, calcium) and one vitamin (B6). For serotonin breakdown, you can see two B vitamins (niacin and riboflavin) as well as one trace mineral (molybdenum). For the two steps involving breakdown of tryptophan, five minerals (calcium, iron, potassium, zinc, copper) and three B vitamins (B1, niacin, and riboflavin) are necessary.

Isn't it amazing how many different nutrients are needed in this tiny section of our brain's metabolic pathways? Four different vitamins and seven different minerals — *eleven micronutrients!* — for optimal function. And since serotonin is so important for our mental health, we all want peak performance of every one of those metabolic steps.

Abridged Tryptophan Metabolism

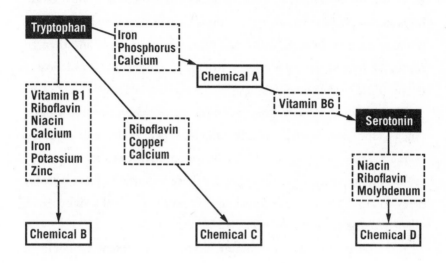

These same types of pathways and metabolic steps are necessary for *all* neurotransmitters, such as dopamine, adrenaline, and GABA, to be manufactured. You are likely realizing by now why it makes perfect sense that a broad spectrum of nutrients is necessary for optimal brain metabolism.

You've likely also realized that all of these nutrients, and others, have to be together. No one nutrient is that special. There is no single magic nutrient to improve brain function. This may seem obvious, but *"Which nutrient should I take to feel better?"* is one of the questions we get asked most often. When that happens, we always say, "That is the wrong question!"

For your brain to perform at its very best, it needs *all* the minerals and vitamins to be swimming through your blood vessels every minute of every day. We'll soon explain what happens when those nutrients are not available to your brain.

Later in this book we will tell you where to find those nutrients, but you can guess that it is not in packaged, ultra-processed food.

Making Energy Molecules

Every cell in our bodies contains multiple tiny structures known as mitochondria. They're the "energy factories" that enable us to live; without them, you would be dead. Mitochondria take in nutrients and then go through lots of steps using those nutrients to produce ATP (adenosine triphosphate) — the energy molecule that is essential for life.

There are many different pieces of the steps involved in this process (such as the Krebs cycle, also called the citric acid cycle, in case you remember this from science class). All that you need to know for now is that everything that drives the sequences of these important cycles is *totally dependent* on dietary nutrients. No one nutrient is essential — they are *all* needed for the cycles to operate.

Nutrients go into the mitochondria, ATP comes out. What could be simpler?

Keeping Your Genes Healthy

The powerful role nutrients play in our health doesn't stop there.

You're probably familiar with the concept of genes or DNA: genes are the bits of chromosome that we inherit from our biological parents. They give us a predisposition to having certain features, or strengths and weaknesses. And maybe you've heard the term "epigenetics"? What does all this have to do with nutrition? Let's take a look.

We are born with a fixed set of genes, but it's important to realize that genes also usually function like a dimmer switch you have on a ceiling light in your home. Genes can be turned *up or down* just like that ceiling light. We refer to that variability as *genetic expression*. But just to be clear, silencing a gene doesn't necessarily mean a trait is *not* expressed (as you will see when we talk about the agouti mouse later in this chapter).

Understanding of genes has really exploded in the last few decades. We've gone from thinking that genes are unmodifiable, to now appreciating that while the genetic code may not change, whether the code is read or not *can* be modified. Consider this: if genes were completely deterministic, clearly and always defining who we are, then identical twins would always have identical strengths and weaknesses. But it has been known for centuries that they do not. Even for diseases or a mental disorder like schizophrenia, the concordance rate (percentage of twins who show identical occurrence) reported by many different studies is less than 80 percent. Admittedly, 80 percent is a very high concordance rate — meaning if your identical twin develops disease X, there is an 80 percent chance that you will too — but the fact that the concordance rate is not fully 100 percent in two individuals with identical genes tells us that there are environmental factors influencing the expression of those genes.

The really interesting question is, what turns your genetic dimmer switches up or down? If you know you might have inherited some genes that can lead to a mental disorder, wouldn't you want to know what to do to modify the expression of those genes?

The biggest category of gene-modifying variables comes from the environment. These environmental factors have been referred to as *epigenetic variables,* or *modifiers of your genes,* ever since the latter half of the twentieth century, when the British scientist C. H. Waddington coined the term.

So how can something like exposure to an environmental factor "boss" our genes around without changing them? One answer is through DNA methylation. Here's a truly amazing fact: *billions* of times every second, your very smart body is transferring atoms in the form of methyl groups (consisting of one carbon and three hydrogen atoms) to your DNA, your hormones, your immune cells, and your neurotransmitters.

This process of creating and transferring methyl groups, known as the methylation cycle, is vital for our health, so we want to make sure it functions at its best. When it does, incredible things happen: little breaks in our DNA that come from wear and tear get repaired! Our hormones are properly regulated! Bits of damage to various cell membranes are healed! And so on.

As you can probably guess, the chemistry behind the production of these methyl groups is well defined, and once again is *dependent on nutrient cofactors*. Lots of different cofactors. Like zinc, folate, vitamin B2, vitamin B6, vitamin B12, and more.

Without an adequate supply of nutrients, methylation will always be impaired. Inadequate dietary intake of these nutrients, nutrient malabsorption, and medications that deplete nutrient levels can all cause methylation imbalances.

Typically, when a gene is methylated it is silenced (the dimmer switch is down), and when it is unmethylated it is more active (dimmer switch is up). In other words, the presence or absence of this methyl group influences whether the DNA will be tightly coiled up so that a gene can't be decoded (or read) or whether it is uncoiled and therefore very readable. Our genes code for proteins, and enzymes are one form of protein. If the genetic code is readable, then those enzymes will be manufactured and can assist with metabolism.

What types of epigenetic variables can influence methylation? The two categories that are most studied are *nutrition* and *environmental toxins*. For example, if you eat a diet of only cookies and chips, your genes probably will not be getting adequate nutrients for methylation to occur optimally. Or, if the air you breathe is polluted or you are a smoker, it can also mess with your genes by switching them on or off through adding or taking away a methyl group, essentially hijacking them.

As you may know, our DNA is subject to hundreds or thousands of "breaks" every day. Exposure to radiation is possibly the best-known cause of many such breaks. What's really neat is that our biology contains many different DNA repair mechanisms; these are systems in place to detect and fix the damage as well as safely dispose of severely damaged cells.

In one fairly dramatic illustration of the importance of nutrition for some of these cellular activities, scientists showed that human cells grown in cultures that lacked folate displayed the same amount and types of DNA breaks that occurred with radiation exposure.[3] Clearly, we have many mechanisms trying to ensure good health, and they all require a plentiful supply of nutrients.

One of the questions that's always asked in any biology class is: "Which is more important — nature or nurture?" This is the same as asking "Which is more important — your genes or your environment?" But it's the wrong question, however it's phrased! The really important question is "How do nature and nurture work together?" Let's look at how this happens for mental health.

Autumn's Inheritance

As you read in the Introduction, Bonnie first heard Autumn's story in 1996, and later she learned that not only had Autumn's mother Debbie died by suicide (described in *A Promise of Hope,* by Autumn Stringam), but that Debbie's father also did. Two generations of suicide and then Autumn's postpartum psychosis made Bonnie decide to interview the family for more information. The result was a three-generation chart showing that in every generation, about 50 percent of the family members had had mental health issues: five out of ten in Autumn's generation, four out of eight in her mother's, and four out of nine in her grandfather's. There was clearly a strong genetic component to Autumn's psychosis—yet the multinutrient supplements had restored Autumn and her siblings to completely normal mental health.

In other words, this family was illustrating exactly what Linus

> Pauling had predicted fifty years ago: a genetic predisposition
> to mental illness was likely caused by a need for more than the
> usual amount of cofactors (minerals and vitamins) to make the
> ideal amount of brain chemicals for those individuals.

Genetics and Mental Health

Ever since the search began in the 1940s for genes related to human health, scientists have also been looking for specific single genes that influence mental health. One of the factors that has propelled that search is the almost universal finding across all cultures that some types of mental disorders do, in fact, run in families. For example, heritability estimates for ADHD are as high as 75 percent. Though family influence can be analyzed in terms of environmental factors, it was long thought that there was some specific gene that could explain the development of psychiatric illnesses that would be discovered someday.

So it makes sense to ask: How has the search for the specific genes for mental disorders been going? Not well.

Over the last few years, there has been a general recognition that the search for specific genes (also called candidate genes) that influence whether a person develops depression or other mental disorders had been pretty much a failure.[4] A May 2019 article in the *Atlantic* by Ed Yong was entitled "A Waste of 1000 Research Papers." Yong wrote that "Decades of early research on the genetics of depression were built on nonexistent foundations. How did that happen?" One of the scientists he interviewed said, "This should be a real cautionary tale . . . How on Earth could we have spent twenty years and hundreds of millions of dollars studying pure noise?"

We think the decades of investment in the search for individual genes may well be analogous to the decades searching for single-nutrient treatments for mental illness, as we will explain. Discovery in science is not a perfect road map, and it is not uncommon for leads to end in dead ends, as it has with the search for candidate genes. Science evolves and can make huge headways from the experience of failure. Fortunately, over the last decade, the search has moved away from candidate genes to looking at the additive effects of *many* gene sites, also known as genome-wide association studies, and this field is showing great promise for discovering the genetic architecture of mental disorders that may someday lead to new treatment options.[5] We hope that nutrition research experiences a similar revolution.

Epigenetics and Mental Health

Are epigenetic effects powerful? Enormously. Honeybees, lab animals, and research with humans can help you understand why.

Honeybees. Honeybees have very complex societies. Only a single queen is fertile and all the rest of the worker bees are sterile. Amazingly, worker bees and queen bees all begin life as genetically identical larvae. What makes them develop into entirely different bees and behave very differently is called a *phenotypic difference*. Even more amazing is that the variable that determines the difference between being the queen bee and being a plain old worker bee is the diet! The colony selects a single larva to be fed a diet high in royal jelly, and that one lucky bee develops ovaries and becomes the queen. Larvae destined to be worker bees are largely fed pollen and nectar (together called beebread), as well as honey.

This worker bee diet contains many plant chemicals that are believed to silence genes by creating changes in DNA methylation; worker bees are literally castrated by their diet. The lucky larva that is fed the royal jelly exclusively not only has its diet enriched, but seems to be protected from the castrating effects of the plant chemicals that appear to modulate gene expression.[6]

How remarkable is that? Using the same genetic hardware, bees have figured out how to use different foods to produce either long-lived reproductive queens or short-lived sterile workers. If anyone thinks nutrition isn't powerful, be sure to tell them about bees!

Lab animals. Since the early part of this century, researchers have been using the yellow agouti mouse model to see if nutritional factors can alter physical appearance and health. They discovered that it is possible to change the coat color, obesity level, and cancer risk in mice, depending on their exposure levels to nutrients such as folate, choline, and vitamin B12.[7] It's a fascinating phenomenon.

All mammals have a gene that's been named *agouti*. When the agouti gene is unmethylated (which results in the gene being expressed), then the mouse will be yellow. If, however, the gene is methylated (and therefore silenced), then the mouse will be its normal brown color. The diet fed to the mother during pregnancy also influences the color of her babies' coats. If she is fed foods that contain micronutrients, like B12 and folate, that are needed to produce methyl groups, then her offspring will be brown. But if the food she eats is low in these nutrients, her offspring might be yellow. Yellow mice might look cute, but they are at higher risk for other health problems.

That is the power of nutrition!

Human physical health. The Framingham Heart Study began in 1948 and has been studying cardiovascular disease in people residing in Framingham, Massachusetts, for decades. In 2019, they reported that in about 5,000 participants, a healthier diet as defined by an index based on adherence to the 2015 American Dietary Guidelines was associated with the expression of genes involved in metabolic function.[8] In other words, the diet seemed to influence whether genes involved in metabolism were silenced or expressed. What is especially relevant is that one particular gene that likely regulates obesity and energy expenditure was found to be moderated by the healthier diet.

We think this is a profoundly important finding in physical health, and that similar discoveries will emerge for brain health in the years to come. Hopefully, we'll soon find the genes that regulate brain metabolism of essential nutrients, which may explain much of mental illness.

Until that happens, what we all need to do is eat better for our brains.

Proof of Concept

As we mentioned, epigenetic DNA modification helps regulate how genes are activated or silenced. DNA changes have been widely implicated in the development of many serious diseases, including cancer, psychiatric disorders, cardiovascular disease, and obesity. Understanding the conditions that contribute to DNA methylation changes, and their implications, is fundamental for development of successful treatments. It is one of the major challenges in human genetics that scientists are facing today.

Along with two genetic collaborators, Drs. Martin Kennedy and Aaron Stevens at the University of Otago, Julia and her team set out to test whether a broad-spectrum multinutrient supplement could lead to DNA methylation changes in children with ADHD. This preliminary study found that yes, it probably can, albeit modestly.

It was the first time nutrient supplementation has been shown to modify genes in humans.[9] The rationale behind this study was that additional nutrients would provide a high quantity of methyl groups that may modify DNA expression. In order to measure any genome-wide changes during the randomized controlled trial (RCT), blood samples were assessed using state-of-the-art technology. The researchers were able to assess DNA methylation at over 850,000 sites in the human genome. This in itself is mind-boggling!

The results showed that multinutrient supplementation did influence DNA methylation, though the magnitude of change is likely quite small, consisting of nonspecific changes that involve several hundred genes. The team concluded that the therapeutic effects of multinutrients are probably not resulting *substantially* from changes in DNA methylation, but the magnitude of the observed changes might increase over time.

Fighting Inflammation

As more and more research shows how excess inflammation causes health problems, we need to point out that equating "unhealthy" with inflammation is incorrect. Inflammation is sometimes good — even life-saving. Every time we're exposed to an infection and our immune system kicks into gear to respond to the invasion of a foreign substance like a virus or bacterium, an inflammatory response is what's needed to fight off the invader. Dr. Andrew Weil explains this so well in his book *Healthy Aging,* when he says that inflammation has "two faces." The positive face is that inflammation is such an important component of our immune systems and our healing processes. The negative face is that excessive ongoing inflammation seems to contribute to many illnesses.

Instead of fighting inflammation, it's much more accurate to say that it's important to fight *excessive* inflammation. Why? It all comes down to a mechanism called homeostasis, which is how our physiology can remain stable. For example, your body works hard to remain at a constant temperature no matter what the weather is.

Our bodies have homeostatic mechanisms to help maintain our levels of inflammation within a restricted range. Your mitochondria play an odd double role in this regard. Creating ATP increases a tiny amount of inflammation — yet ATP is one of our best weapons against excessive inflammation, too. This is one very complicated homeostatic mechanism!

The really puzzling thing is that so many of the studies on inflammation and health conclude with a discussion of drug development. Their message is that we need to develop anti-inflammatory pharmaceuticals to fight excessive inflammation. That is certainly a valid message in some ways, as anti-inflammatory meds play an important role in various health problems such as arthritis. But let's not forget about the extensive use of anti-inflammatory *diets*, an approach first pioneered in the 1930s for heart disease.

Protecting Yourself from Environmental Toxins

We are often asked if environmental pollutants are contributing to the epidemic of mental health problems. There are some links being reported in relation to toxins for both mental and neurodevelopmental disorders.

To study some of these questions, Bonnie was awarded a large grant in 2008 to track a group of 2,200 pregnant women to study nutrition during pregnancy and later. She brought together an interdisciplinary group of about fifteen scientists with expertise in obstetrics, family medicine, nutrition, neurodevelopment, genetics, developmental disorders, and mental health, and they named their study APrON (Alberta Pregnancy Outcomes and Nutrition).[10] Although Bonnie stepped down as team leader to retire in 2016, the study continues to flourish with many additional scientists and spinoff studies (ApronStudy.ca).

For example, remember the worldwide concern that surfaced a few years ago about bisphenol A found in baby bottles? BPA is an industrial chemical used in the manufacture of plastics. The vast majority of us have detectable levels of BPA in our urine, due to exposure to plastics, to thermal receipts, and even from some of our food. Studies from around the world have shown strong evidence of a relationship between prenatal exposure to BPA and increased risk of neurodevelopmental problems in children, such as poorer motor skills, and problems with attention, hyperactivity, and social communication.[11]

The APrON scientists studied BPA in a subgroup of ninety-eight mother-child pairs.[12] Urine samples were taken from the mothers during their second trimester of pregnancy, and then later from their children when they were three to five years old. The children were also studied with a type of brain scan called diffusion tensor imaging (DTI), which provides information about white matter microstructure. They found that the level of BPA in the *maternal* second-trimester urine samples was associated with brain microstructure changes in their three-to-five-year-old children, particularly less developed areas in white matter tracts (those are the myelin sheaths around the axons, or fibers, of neurons). In addition, the DTI results were associated with children having more of what are called internalizing behaviors — anxiety, depression, social withdrawal, and physical complaints — when they were three to five years old.

One of the implications of this line of research relates to children's ability to cope with stress. In 132 mother-infant pairs from APrON, maternal urine samples collected during the second trimester were analyzed for total BPA, and then when their infants were six weeks old, infant emotional reactivity was evaluated when they were poked for a blood sample.[13] They found that an increase in prenatal BPA exposure might mediate increased stress reactivity of the infants, but only in males. (This sex difference might seem random, but it's well supported in animal research, too.) In other words, *exposure to plastics during pregnancy can affect the ability to regulate emotions,* especially for males. Further research is being carried out to determine how nutrition may buffer potential harms of exposure to toxins such as plastics for children.

Another group of chemicals that are of great concern are phthalates, used to make plastics soft and pliable, as well as in many self-care products such as deodorants and baby powder. APrON scientists also published data showing that prenatal levels of phthalates are associated with changes in brain white matter microstructure, and may underlie both internalizing and externalizing behavior problems.[14] These studies are very concerning and warrant further study into the effects of toxins, so we can see how to better protect infant brain development. And nutrition is likely an important protective factor. In laboratory animals, it has already been known for many years that nutrient supplementation *protects* against some of the effects of BPA.[15]

In 2012 an important review of nutrition as a buffer for environmental pollutants was published in *Environmental Health Perspectives*.[16] It concluded that what we eat is such an important modulator of toxicity from environmental chemicals that dietary information needs to be included in all assessments of risk. They proposed that poor dietary habits increase our vulnerability to environmental chemicals — not just in the short term, but through life. In contrast, a diet rich in antioxidants and other anti-inflammatory nutrients may reduce that vulnerability. Early intervention as well as teaching people about the protective effects of nutrition is in the best interests of all our countries struggling to control the environmental and chemical pollutants plaguing their citizens.

These five examples of systems in the body that need a broad spectrum of nutrients help us understand why we need to eat a variety of foods. That's the only way to get the variety of nutrients for optimal brain function. It's no surprise that Mother Nature has provided them to us all together, and in proper balance, especially in fruits and vegetables!

When Does Your Brain Need *More* Nutrients?

Now that you know how important nutrients are for regular management of your brain function, let's think about all those times when your brain may need more nutrients than usual.

When Dealing with Acute and Chronic Stress:
The Triage Theory

Stress is an inevitable part of life and exacerbates any health problem. Yet as stated in the quotation at the top of this chapter, it is unlikely that stress is the *primary* cause of any mental health problem. Instead, it is the *lack of resilience* that is a major contributor to illness. As you'll see in chapter 7, improving your nutrient intake should be your go-to method for improving your resilience.

Our bodies have incredible mechanisms that enable one system to override others at any given time, depending on circumstances. Favoring one bodily system over another in a crisis is called the triage theory.

Think about this as you would if you had the misfortune to be sitting at the triage station in an emergency room. Even if you are sure you have broken your ankle, a more severely ill or injured patient will always be treated first. The same thing happens with our bodies. Managing the fight/flight response always trumps all other functions.

You already know about the triage theory if, when you were a child, your parents sternly warned you to wait thirty minutes after eating before going swimming. That was all about bodily systems and which one takes precedence — because when you eat, your digestive system directs blood flow away from the muscles in your limbs and toward the stomach and intestines. For that period of time after eating, your gut needs blood more than your legs and arms do, which is why your parents worried you might get a cramp while swimming.

You also know about triage if you learned that in pregnant women, blood flow and nutrients are prioritized to favor the baby. The fetus gets fed first if there are limited resources, because it is highly vulnerable.

When we get stressed, our bodies automatically click into fight/flight mode. When stress becomes chronic, our bodies react by keeping that fight/flight response in constant activation — and this can lead to chronic nutrient depletion. Just think about the barrage of "threats" that exist in our daily lives — work pressures, traffic jams, the kids having meltdowns after a long day at school, and financial woes. Even worrying about existential threats, like climate change or pandemic viruses, can rob our bodies of nutrients.

The fight/flight response has evolved to ensure our survival as a species, so it will always take precedence in terms of getting access to nutrients first. But all of these modern-day threats activate the fight/flight response and keep it activated, leading to excessive release of the stress hormones, adrenaline and cortisol.

While you need these hormones to help you manage acute stress as it is occurring, *chronic* stress is a different story. The consequences of relentless stress over the long haul could explain why they lead to problems with mood and anxiety regulation, sleep, and poor concentration. Nature ensures that the nutrient-dependent functions you need for short-term survival (like the fight/flight response) are protected at the expense of longer-term functions (like concentration).

Fortunately, the way to replenish the empty fuel tank and mitigate chronic stress is by doing something that is under your control: giving yourself the additional nutrients you need.

When There Are Genetic Differences, or
Inborn Errors of Metabolism

You already know how important nutrients are for optimal brain metabolism. Without sufficient amounts, all of the metabolic pathways in your brain can become slow and inefficient.

But some people also have what's called an inborn error of metabolism associated with a defective enzyme that results in needing a larger-than-normal amount of nutrients to work. This isn't an entirely new concept: we've known about this in relation to physical health for at least two decades. In 2002, leading American biochemist Bruce Ames summarized fifty human genetic mutations causing an excessively high need for certain vitamin cofactors to make enzymes work, and there are probably many additional mutations associated with mineral cofactors.[17] Each of the syndromes Ames described resulted in a known physical ailment, and each one could be corrected by giving the patients additional vitamins to optimize their enzymatic reactions and make them more efficient. These syndromes are ones with long unfamiliar biochemical names, such as branched chain alpha-ketoacid dehydrogenase, associated with intellectual disability and ataxia. But the point is, this phenomenon is proven in physical health — some people are genetically programmed to need more micronutrients than others for their metabolic pathways to work efficiently, and giving that individual a large amount of the vitamins ameliorates the problem.

Even though the brain is the most metabolically demanding organ in your body, it tends to be overlooked when investigating whether or not it has "sluggish pathways" — or inefficient brain metabolism. Some people might inherit the kind of genetic differences that mean they need *more* nutrients than others. If they don't know this — and right now it is impossible to test for, in the area of mental disorders — their pathways might be slower, leading to less-than-excellent brain function.

Why does this matter? As you know, neurotransmitters are the brain chemicals that enable neurons to communicate with each other. They go through many metabolic steps involving their synthesis, uptake, and breakdown. Each of those steps requires enzymes . . . and every enzyme needs multiple cofactors to do the work. Zinc, for example, is essential for at least a hundred enzyme systems, and it is only one of the approximately fifteen minerals required by your brain.

Wouldn't it be amazing if this phenomenon explained some mental symptoms too?

"Metabolic" Genes and Mental Health — the MTHFR Gene

There are, in fact, a few genes already identified that could be related to brain metabolism. MTHFR (methylenetetrahydrofolate reductase) is the one mentioned most in mental health, although there are others — notably CBS and BHMT (each involved in metabolic steps converting homocysteine into glutathione and methionine, respectively) and COMT (involved in the breakdown of neurotransmitters like dopamine, noradrenaline, and adrenaline) — but MTHFR is definitely the one we get asked about the most. To get an idea of how popular this gene is, a Google search for MTHFR gave 2,770,000 hits!

What is so important about MTHFR? The MTHFR gene codes for the MTHFR enzyme. If an individual inherits a version of MTHFR that causes less of that enzyme to be manufactured, then the methylation cycle *may* not work so well. This is actually quite common. But, since the role of nutrients is to function as cofactors for enzymes, flooding those enzymes with nutrients — like folate that is already methylated (called methylfolate) — can speed up the metabolic reaction to near-normal function.

There's a lot of hype about the importance of different genes, and sometimes this hype is out of proportion to the published data. Suffice to say for now that MTHFR is just *one* gene coding for *one* enzyme out of thousands and thousands of enzymes that your body uses. When websites recommend you invest your money to determine which variation of MTHFR you have, they are giving you the impression that this is a magic bullet gene! With rare exceptions, this is simply not the case. With MTHFR, the research is incredibly variable — for example, in Julia's research, she did not find more of these MTHFR "variants" in kids with ADHD compared to the general population, and presence or absence of the variant did not predict response to nutrients.[18] This lack of any substantial finding should not surprise you, given what we told you about the wasted search for single genes!

As we have often been told by our geneticist colleagues, there is no medical reason to test these common variants as there are no recommended actions based on the results of such genetic tests.

When You Are Taking Certain Medications Long Term

Millions of medications are prescribed every day for long-term use. Not just for psychiatric conditions, but for high blood pressure, heart disease, diabetes, inflammatory diseases, digestive issues, and to prevent pregnancy.

If you are prescribed any medication for long-term use, you should always read up on potential long-term effects. That's not always easy. In fact, many of these meds can cause you to need *more* nutrients to counter their side effects over time, but you probably won't be told about that in the leaflet that comes with your prescription.

If you knew where to look up the research on the interaction between nutrients and medications, you would find a lot of studies and summaries about how medication use can interfere with nutrient status.[19] Here are just a few, so you can see how common it is for medications to reduce the nutrient supply for the brain:

Aspirin can negatively affect vitamin C levels.

Contraceptives can decrease folate, magnesium, and vitamins B6, C, and E.

Metformin, commonly prescribed for pre-diabetes, weight management, and metabolic disorders, can reduce vitamin B12.

Mood stabilizers can reduce folic acid, vitamin D, vitamin B6, and vitamin B12 levels, as well as minerals such as copper, selenium, and zinc.

Proton pump inhibitors lower the production of gastric acid in your stomach, but they also can decrease absorption of micronutrients that depend on low pH for uptake into the intestinal cells, such as B12, calcium, zinc, and magnesium.

Statins. A quarter of American women and men over the age of forty take a statin![20] But statins can inhibit the function of CoQ10, an essential player in the citric acid cycle, which is so important for production of our energy molecule ATP.

You need to be aware that these life-saving drugs may have inadvertent side effects that could affect your brain health.

But there is also good news. Increasing your nutrient supply may reverse the depletion caused by these medications. Even better, more nutrients might also help you lower the dose of some prescriptions, as you'll read about in chapter 5.

When Fighting Excess Inflammation

Another factor that can lead to a need for more nutrients is excessive, chronic inflammation. There are plenty of stressors like environmental toxins and bad food choices that can cause excessive inflammation. What can be done to keep inflammation in check? As usual, the answer is partly about what you eat. An anti-inflammatory diet is high in the micronutrients and phytonutrients (plant-based nutrients) that are so critical for balancing the inflammatory factors in our lives.

Antioxidants are one of the ways to reduce this excessive inflammation. Glutathione, a small protein based on three amino acids, is an especially powerful antioxidant, and is the end product of one of the pathways in the methylation cycle. So it isn't surprising that there are researchers trying to determine if giving more of the B vitamins needed for production of glutathione by the methylation cycle results in reduced inflammation.

When Pregnant

Many of the countless millions of pregnant women in the world do not have access to or don't take enough prenatal vitamin and mineral supplements, which can help protect developing fetuses from common birth defects. And supplementing with these nutrients isn't just for the baby, but also for the overall health of expectant mothers, to reduce their long-term risk for illness, ensure the best outcome for the infant, and reduce birth complications, risk of preeclampsia, and likelihood of postnatal depression.[21]

Many studies have shown how common it is for pregnant women to be eating enough calories, but not enough essential fatty acids, vitamins, and minerals.[22] In the APrON group of women described earlier in this chapter, there was a significant relationship between what the women ate in terms of vitamin D content and what their blood levels showed, but the bottom line was that their intake from both diet and supplements together was not enough to give them the desired levels in their blood.[23] In other words, even this group of women who were above average in terms of education and economic status did not meet government recommendations for ideal vitamin D levels during pregnancy.

There are other studies with findings consistent with APrON's data relating prenatal nutrition to childhood behavior. For instance, as described in chapter 4, a number of studies looking at mother-child pairs have found that a higher intake of food low in nutrient content predicted behavioral problems in the children up to the age of eight; however, exposure to toxins was not examined in any of those studies. Considering the role of nutrition as a protection against environmental toxins is an important focus for future studies.

Since pregnancy is a life stage where the demand for nutrients increases substantially, expectant mothers should always adjust their nutrient intake accordingly. For women who live in poverty or who don't have regular access to highly nutritious food, this can be a daunting task. Many of the recipes we provide in chapter 9 are less expensive than ultra-processed foods.

During Adolescence

Another metabolically active time is during the teenage years. Essentially, during this stage of development, the brain undergoes huge growth, forming new wiring and new connections, especially in the frontal lobes that are in charge of cognitive skills, impulsivity, and emotional regulation. If you've lived with a teenager, you likely were astonished by how much food these kids could pack away without becoming overweight.

Anyone who has raised or regularly interacted with teenagers also knows that these years can be a bit fraught! It's not just due to the hormonal changes these kids are going through, but the fact that *their brains are currently under construction,* as Julia is fond of saying about her two teenaged sons. It might be a bit easier to manage (or ignore!) their behavior when you realize the enormous development of their brains that they're enduring, while also appreciating that their need for nutrients is much greater.

The latest news about adolescent eating habits is slightly positive, but still well below the ideal. A report on dietary intake from more than 30,000 youth aged 2 to 19, extracted from the United States National Health and Nutrition Examination Survey cycles covering 1999–2016, categorized people's diets as poor, intermediate, or ideal based on how they compared to American Heart Association standards.[24] Overall, improvements labeled as "modest" by the authors were detectable over the seventeen years, but the diets of two-thirds of those in their teen years were still categorized as poor in 2016.

During the Aging Process

The focus of this book is on *mental* health, but of course this topic is an essential component of overall *brain* health. We are often asked about aging and dementia by friends and colleagues, so we closely monitor the relevant research. Clearly, the results are following a path that is parallel to mental health: no single nutrient can protect us from dementia, but a better diet and broader spectrum of micronutrients seem to help (as you'll learn in chapters 6 and 8).

Some of this research draws from many years of basic science showing that we lose some of our ability to mitigate the effects of oxidative stress (the naturally occurring imbalance between free radicals and anti-oxidants in your body) as we age. Obviously, many researchers are trying to find ways to slow down the aging process. Back in the 1990s, there were many studies showing that laboratory rats given higher doses of nutrients exhibited improvements on a broad variety of measures indicative of re-versed aging, such as improved antioxidant protection, increased neu-rotransmitter function, and better learning ability.[25]

In the ensuing decades, has this information been applied to *human* brain health? The answer is a very strong yes. But, as with the research on mental health, the media coverage and physician information still focus on pharmaceutical treatments, even though *no single drug treatment* has been proven effective for cognitive decline — a term we use to refer to mild cognitive impairment and all forms of dementia including Alzheim-er's. Some meds do provide some relief of symptoms, but not one can halt the inevitable progress of declining cognition.

The right amount of nutrients can, however, reduce some of the factors that speed up the aging process. A 2019 study questioned nearly 200,000 individuals with no cognitive impairment initially, and who were catego-rized as being at high, intermediate, or low genetic risk for dementia.[26] Even in those with a high genetic risk, a favorable lifestyle that included a healthy diet was associated with a lower risk of developing dementia an average of eight years later.

Nutrients and antioxidant foods (such as blueberries) are vital for fighting the adverse effects of aging.[27] We'll review some of these ideas in later chapters.

One mechanism by which nutrients might protect against cognitive decline is by protecting telomere length. Telomeres are the DNA se-quences at the ends of all our chromosomes, and they are a biomarker of aging: shorter telomeres are associated with a shortened life expectancy.

Chronic stress, a poor diet, oxidative stress, and inflammation accelerate the loss of our telomeres, a process called attrition.[28] Scientists Elizabeth Blackburn and Elissa Epel from the University of California, San Francisco, in their book *The Telomere Effect*, clearly explained the types of things that wear down our telomeres and shorten our lives: chronic stress, processed food diet, exposure to environmental toxins, and so on. In support of that information, a cross-sectional analysis of 886 older adults participating in the SUN project in Spain (Seguimiento Universidad de Navarra) found that those who reported eating the most ultra-processed food had the shortest telomeres.[29] The antioxidant type of diet shown to protect telomere length is going to sound very familiar to you when you read about the type of diet we recommend for mental health!

Some of the most important research has come from the laboratory of the late Professor Martha Clare Morris. In her book *Diet for the MIND*, she explained the relationship between what you eat and cognitive decline. This led to the development of what she called the MIND Diet: Mediterranean-DASH Intervention for Neurodegenerative Delay; DASH refers to the Dietary Approach to Stop Hypertension concept promoted by the National Institutes of Health.

The MIND diet is an excellent pathway to achieve brain health, with basic principles similar to what you'll find in chapter 8. Several studies had shown the association between a MIND type of diet and slowed progression toward dementia, and then a four-and-a-half-year study of almost a thousand individuals revealed about a 50 percent reduction in risk for dementia in those who followed a Mediterranean diet most closely.[30] Amazingly, those who carefully followed the MIND diet were identified as being 7.5 years cognitively "younger" than those who didn't follow the diet.[31]

Nutrition and cognitive decline is still a woefully under-recognized topic. Part of the problem is that our ability to absorb nutrients may decrease with age, particularly if digestive acidity decreases, which is a very common trajectory. In that case, several nutrients in particular, such as folic acid, vitamin B12, calcium, iron, and beta carotene, may not be absorbed well.[32] You can see why, as we get older, we may well need more nutrients than we did in our twenties!

The Takeaway

1. Nutrients are absolutely critical in at least five ways: to build your brain and enable your built brain to function, to make energy molecules, to modulate your DNA expression and keep your genes healthy, to fight inflammation, and to protect you from toxins. For daily operation of your brain, nutrients are the fundamental building blocks, making neurotransmitters, supporting the methylation process, and ensuring adequate ATP production. And with adequate ATP production, we are able to repair the various types of chromosomal breaks that occur as a function of environmental stressors.

2. There is good reason to believe that some psychiatric symptoms can be the result of metabolic dysfunction—which is caused when you don't have enough vitamin and mineral cofactors to meet your brain's metabolic needs.

3. Some people might inherit genetic differences that make them need more nutrients than others for optimal brain function. Raising these nutrient levels can have an amazing effect on neurotransmitters and brain health. When that happens, in some cases medication is no longer needed for complete control of mental health symptoms. If you feel particularly vulnerable because of your family background, enhance your nutrient intake. We'll show you how to do that

in chapters 8 and 11, but in the meantime, know that genetic expression is modifiable and nutrients should be one of your go-to tools.

4. Nutrition can and should be the first line of defense you turn to for combating excessive inflammation and the toxic effects of environmental pollution. It should also be at the top of your list when you take certain medications, are pregnant, are suffering from higher levels of stress than usual, and are just getting older!

5. There is no single magic nutrient! All nutrients are important for optimal brain health. Although many other lifestyle factors like exercise and a satisfying emotional life are important, it is absolutely essential to feed your brain all the nutrients it needs for excellent metabolism. This is what will optimize your mental health. As we often say in our lectures, nutrients are *foundational* for healthy brain function.

3

NOT YOUR GRANDMOTHER'S PEACH: FACTORS THAT HAVE LED TO DECREASED NUTRIENT INTAKE

All diseases begin in the gut.

— HIPPOCRATES (C. 460–C. 370 BCE)

DO YOU KNOW WHY phrases like "gut feelings," "gut instinct," "butter-flies in my stomach," "gut-wrenching," "gutsy move," "feeling gutted" are so popular? Because our emotional language revolves around our guts! We're going to show you how these ancient phrases are based in solid science. Even though being able to identify and sequence the DNA of the little organisms living in your gut is a relatively new development, we've known intuitively for a long time that the gut is linked to the function of your brain.

The World of Microbiomes

One of the most astonishing facts about the human body is that at least 50 percent of the cells that live in and on our bodies are not *human* cells, containing human DNA.[1] Instead, these cells are made up of microbes (tiny microorganisms like bacteria) — which leads to a mind-bending question: Are we serving them or are they serving us?

Unless we care for these microbes well, we can sicken and even die. So it's very important to know how these microbes help us, and how we should feed and care for them properly.

A microbiome is a community of microorganisms, such as bacteria, viruses, or fungi, that live together. We speak of the *oral microbiome* to refer to the various microbes living in our mouths. We have a *skin microbiome*, a *stomach microbiome*, a *colon microbiome*, women have a *vaginal microbiome*, and there are many others. Your gut is the biggest — it contains about 90 percent of the microbes in your body.

Each of these microbiomes can be broken down into much more specialized communities. For instance, in the *oral microbiome*, the microbes that live on your tongue are different from the ones in your cheeks. And even more specialization exists: the microbes that live on your teeth *above* the gumline are different from the ones that live *under* the gumline. There are other astonishing specializations as well; some communities of microbes that exist in your eyelashes differ from those on other hairy areas of your body!

In addition, the soil in which we grow our food has its own microbiome. This is an entirely different and crucial population of microbes, which we'll discuss in the second half of this chapter.

There are some basic principles, or descriptors, that are relevant to microbiomes wherever they are found:

- *Diversity is generally good.* Every microbiome, when healthy, contains billions of microbes of many different types. Diversity can be affected by several variables like age — the older we are, the less diverse our microbiomes.[2]
- *Humans have become efficient microbial murderers.* In the past seventy

years or so, we humans have become quite expert at killing microbes. To get rid of microbes in and on our bodies, we use antibiotics and antiseptics, even though antibiotic use with infants can have a profound effect on long-term health.[3] In the soil, we use pesticides and herbicides. They all do the same thing: decrease the microbial population.

- *Dysbiosis* is the general term sometimes used to describe an unbalanced microbiome, wherever it occurs. When we use something to kill off some "problem" microbes that are making us sick, we inevitably disturb the natural, healthy balance of the microbial community.

- *Many of the microorganisms that naturally colonize a healthy body help us.* Some of the ways they do this can be by synthesizing vitamins, or by working with our immune system. Unfortunately, when we take an antibiotic, especially one described as broad-spectrum, many of the good bugs are killed off along with the bad bugs, and you can end up with diarrhea or other stomach problems as a result.

- *To maintain good health, microbiomes need to be properly fed.* Whether we're talking about our gut microbiome or the soil microbiome required for growing our food, the organisms should be fed what they need. People need to be fed plants with a broad spectrum of minerals, vitamins, and other nutrients. Soil needs to be fed a broad spectrum of minerals so that it can grow healthy and nutritious plants.

Intestinal Health and the Gut Microbiome

The trillions of microbes that inhabit the human digestive tract represent the vast majority of nonhuman cells in and on our bodies. So we need to pay a lot of attention to the gut microbiome simply because of its dominance. Just remember that the digestive process starts the second you put any food or drink in your mouth. As Cass Nelson-Dooley points out in her 2019 book *Heal Your Oral Microbiome*, we swallow 140 billion bacterial cells every day, basically helping to seed our intestinal microbiome.

She refers to the mouth and the gut as being "just two stops on the same bus line," so it's not surprising that the major bacteria found in adults, the *Bacteroidetes* and the *Firmicutes,* are in both the oral and the intestinal microbiomes. In both locations, these microbes thrive on a plant-based diet. Eating plants is one of the best ways to benefit your microbiome.

In addition to playing a crucial role in digesting food, the intestinal microbes play pivotal roles in immune and metabolic functioning as well as gene expression, and they may even influence mental health.[4] When your microbiome gets unbalanced, you may know it if you get physical symptoms like reflux, pain, constipation, and/or diarrhea. Dysbiosis is also thought to cause increased permeability of the gut wall — what's now commonly referred to as "leaky gut."

Basically, if you do have a leaky gut caused by inflammation and a lowered ability to utilize the nutrients you're eating, various molecules that should remain in the gut can move outward. When this happens, inflammatory microbes are released into the bloodstream — which is precisely where you don't want them to be. This seems to be a mechanism by which poor gut health can lead to brain dysfunction.

The Direction of Causality Was Probably Going the Wrong Way!

In the 1980s, studies reported that most patients treated in mental health clinics said they suffered with stomachaches, indigestion, diarrhea, and/or constipation. Interestingly, the interpretation of those studies always assumed that the mental health problem was the *cause,* and the dysbiosis was the *effect.* In other words, the investigators thought they proved that feeling depressed or anxious gave people tummyaches. When, much more likely, they had it backwards!

The current explosion of interest in the microbiome looks at the exact opposite direction of causality — that digestive problems may be one cause of mental health problems. If this is correct, then changing the health of the gut microbiome could have significant implications for mental function.

Implications for Mental Health

Although research on the human microbiome has grown exponentially in the past decade, it was only recently that we could identify and describe the bugs within our microbiome in detail. We can now identify bacterial diversity, as well as details about the specific family (e.g., *Bifidobacteriaceae*), genus (e.g., *Bifidobacterium*), and species (e.g., *Bifidobacterium longum*). What scientists are now wondering is whether our gut bugs can change how we *feel*. Can they make us impulsive or depressed? And if so, if we change these microbes, could we become less impulsive or a lot happier? Can a better diet help you do that?

Some patients with certain intestinal infections can have a very hard time getting rid of these bugs, which are increasingly antibiotic-resistant. They can even die. A process called a fecal microbiota transplant implants healthy feces from a donor into the infected gut, and patients who had been very sick can make a full recovery. (For more, see the section "Fecal Microbiota Transplant" later in this chapter.)

If bacteria from a healthy person's gut microbiome can eliminate physical infections, maybe they could change mental health conditions, too. There is very interesting research in laboratory animals to support the idea that changing gut bacteria can change behavior. In one remarkable study, when mice developed by scientists as a model of ASD had their gut microbes changed to ones more typical of normal mice, their autistic-like behaviors improved.[5]

Other research has found substantial evidence that certain emotional traits (like anxiety) could be transferred between different mice! How was that done? By transferring gut microbes from one mouse to another.[6] Even more amazing was what happened when gut bugs from mice who seemed to be anxious were transferred to mice who were more gregarious. The gregarious mice became more anxious. In addition, the levels of an important brain chemical, BDNF (brain-derived neurotrophic factor), found in the hippocampus — a brain area closely associated with emotions like anxiety — decreased. And the opposite also took place: gut bugs from the gregarious mice transferred into the anxious mice caused their anxiety levels to go down and their BDNF levels to go up.[7]

This is direct evidence that when you change the intestinal microbiome, you can also change brain function. Scientists believe that there are a number of communication channels through which the microbiome can influence neural pathways in the brain, including changes in immunity, metabolism, and endocrine function.[8] The vagus nerve, which controls the parasympathetic nervous system and is responsible for much of the communication between the gut and the brain, also plays a role in the regulation of emotional responses.[9] It literally tells your brain how you're feeling — which is why you can trust your "gut feeling"! This may explain why a less diverse microbiome is associated with poor mental health status.[10] There is also research implicating the microbiome in causing teen distress[11] and child misbehavior.[12]

Some research also suggests that specific bacterial strains are associated with specific disorders, like ADHD, schizophrenia, and depression, but the results of these studies have so far been mixed, so we can't confidently say whether a strain is "good" or "bad."[13] There is even research that has identified that certain microbes (*Coprococcus* and *Dialister*) are completely missing in people who are depressed.[14] Whether this absence is a cause of the depression, or whether the cause is the treatment, or whether some other variables are involved, has yet to be determined. It may turn out to be that what matters most is a ratio or a specific concentration of certain strains rather than their presence or absence.

Unfortunately, we're not at a stage yet where we can define a healthy gut microbiome for optimal brain function. Even if you got your own gut microbiome analyzed, it's too soon to know which strains could correct any specific mental health problem. Hopefully this will change in the future.

Treatments That Can Change Your Microbiome

Even though we don't know what makes a perfect microbiome, research that focuses on different treatments is rapidly expanding, with new studies out every week. Scientists are trying to find new ways to improve health through changing the diet (eating more fibrous prebiotics), adding in bacteria (in the form of probiotics), fecal transplants, or micronutrient supplementation. All of these methods are aimed at reversing the dysbiosis that is caused by the nutrient-poor Western diet that is primarily based on ultra-processed foods.[15] Which means, of course, that the easiest and absolute first step to improving your gut health is to improve your diet!

Prebiotic Foods

Did you know that you need to feed the good bugs that are working for you in your gut? Fortunately, a whole foods diet full of prebiotics does just that.

A prebiotic is a nondigestible type of dietary fiber, found in specific types of plant-based foods, that feeds gut bacteria. This is beneficial for the population and activity of your gut microbes. Prebiotics can also enhance immunity, increase absorption of minerals, and induce production of anti-inflammatory compounds.

Sounds great, but the treatment implications are not yet clear. A meta-analysis — one that pools together many studies — of people who didn't have mental health problems found *no* effect of prebiotics on depression and anxiety.[16] There's been only one study targeting people who were clinically depressed, and that, too, showed that the prebiotics studied had *no* effect on depression levels.[17]

More studies are being conducted, and it is certainly possible that the research will catch up to what seems like a good idea — feed your bacteria well and you will be healthy. And even if prebiotics turn out to have absolutely no effect on mental health, every time you eat fibrous plant foods, your gut bacteria produce butyric acid, which is very important for the health of your gut lining. That's one of the reasons why eating a heavily processed diet, where the fiber has been removed from your food, is so bad for you. The more processed, the less fiber. So make sure your diet includes beans, lentils, asparagus, onions, garlic, leeks, and beets. These are all foods that are naturally rich in prebiotics.

What About Probiotics?

Probiotics are now stacked on shelves in drugstores all over the world, with claims that they can treat all kinds of ailments — from irritable bowel syndrome to diarrhea to stress to low mood. It's taken many years for this supplementation to become well known and well used, however. Bonnie remembers reading an article in the 1970s describing the Russian medical practice of always prescribing probiotics for patients who needed to take antibiotics. That practice seemed to be unheard of in North America. However, back then, there was a theory (never really proven) that the reason for the unusual longevity of people in countries like Azerbaijan and Georgia was that they ate a lot of yogurt. Keep in mind that the homemade yogurt that these healthy old folks consumed had little in common with the heavily sweetened yogurts that most Westerners eat!

The media has jumped all over probiotics, even implying that they're the next best thing to prescription antidepressants, with headlines like "Are Probiotics the New Prozac?" or "Could Bacteria Be the Answer to Treating Depression?"

Many of these headlines actually come from studies conducted on *healthy* young adults. For example, the study with the first direct proof that probiotics can affect brain function in healthy humans compared the brain activity of forty-six women, some who had consumed a fermented milk product with beneficial bacteria over a four-week period, some who had consumed a placebo, and some who had received no intervention.[18] Based on functional magnetic resonance imaging (fMRI—a type of brain scan), those who'd been given the fermented drink showed greater activity in the regions of their brains that control central processing of emotion and sensation than the placebo group.

There have now been dozens of clinical trials investigating how well probiotics can treat psychiatric conditions. Most are focused on mood, but some have been done on anxiety and autism. The overall message is mixed, and while there appears to be an effect, it is likely modest.[19] Having said that, the effect appears to be larger in people who suffer from depression, compared to those without depression. And the bugs in the running for the most evidence seem to be from the *Bifidobacterium* and *Lactobacillus* genus.

The idea that supplemented probiotic bacteria could be used as a treatment for depression is a fairly recent one. The term "psychobiotics" was coined by psychiatrist Ted Dinan and neuroscientist John Cryan to describe probiotic bacteria that produce health benefits in patients suffering from mental health problems.[20] Many other reviews extol the virtues of probiotics and their potential for reducing inflammation and improving brain function. Animal models have also shown that taking probiotics can affect emotional behavior. This might be due to their ability to alter the microbial composition of the gut, how they can limit the production of pro-inflammatory cytokines (proteins important in cell signaling), and how they can reduce inflammation. All of this can have a positive effect on gut-brain communication.[21]

You might also want to consider using probiotics as prevention, and not just treatment. An amazing study gave babies either probiotics (*Lactobacillus rhamnosus*) or a placebo, and then followed up *thirteen* years later to see if any of them had ADHD or autism.[22] ADHD or autism were diagnosed in 17 percent of the children in the placebo group — and *none* in the probiotic group. That's a pretty strong effect, and we hope researchers are going to keep on studying this potentially powerful prevention.

But there are two fundamental problems with all the probiotic supplement research. The first is that most of the studies are conducted on healthy people. And the second is that the researchers all have their favorite bacteria. Some use *Lactobacillus casei* and others use *bifidobacterium bifidum* or *lactobacillus helveticus*. And then some combine two or three of these strains as well as others, which means it is harder to know what effect a specific strain is having on health. Doing a meta-analysis — which some scientists love to do — ends up comparing apples and oranges, and showing a weak effect overall.

So what does this mean? Well, like most anything, the craze seems to come before the evidence. We need to be a little more cautious about believing that probiotics are going to help alleviate psychological symptoms, especially as we really have no way to know which strains are best, what the optimal dose is, how long the intervention needs to be, whether the bugs listed on a label are really present, or even if they get into our guts. Much more research is needed. Many people do sometimes get better on probiotics — they just don't often get greater benefit than the placebo group. The best way to consume probiotics? From your food! A good place to start would be unsweetened yogurt and fermented foods like kimchi, sauerkraut, or kombucha.

Julia vividly remembers one woman in her sixties, with a long history of "treatment-resistant" depression, who was enrolled in a probiotic study, run by a former student of Julia's, Dr. Amy Romijn, who was evaluating the effects of two bacterial strains on symptoms of depression. One day, this woman saw Julia in her lab, and the woman came running up to her, full of energy, giving Julia an enormous hug and kiss and thanking her profusely for changing her life. Later, they found out she was on the placebo. This is how powerful the placebo effect can be!

One very important feature of the probiotic research that will have to be addressed is the number and quantity of bacterial strains. Often, when we write about nutrients, or even medications, we mention the importance of the dose — meaning how much you need to take. But in the probiotic world, there are dozens of strains, and each one might have different effects at different dosage levels. Are some more important than others? We still don't know.

We do worry a bit that this search for some magic bullet, problem-solving set of bacteria may turn out to be disappointing, but it is worth some effort to figure out if this is an important lead. It is an exciting time and a field to follow closely.

Fecal Microbiota Transplant (FMT)

As you read earlier in this chapter, a fecal microbiota transplant takes place when a sample of the microbiome of a healthy donor is given to an unhealthy patient. This is usually done during a colonoscopy, or sometimes via capsules (yup — crapsules). Although the thought of it might make you feel a bit squeamish, this process was developed to save lives, and it has a remarkable success rate.

FMT is also called a stool transplant, gut flora transplant, microbiota transfer therapy, or bacteriotherapy. It actually has a long history, with the first documented use by Ge Hong, a Chinese physician who, in the fourth century, gave it in the form of a broth to patients with severe diarrhea caused by food poisoning. Although likely used quite widely at the time, FMT was then forgotten about for centuries. It reemerged as a treatment in the 1950s, when it was used at a hospital in Denver to treat four patients with severe *Clostridium difficile* (*C. diff*) infection who were not expected to survive. Within twenty-four hours of FMT, all four patients had fully recovered.[23]

These data are pretty remarkable, with more recent research showing that FMT successfully treated over 80 percent of recurrent *C. diff* infections, making it a standard treatment.[24] There aren't very many treatments able to claim that success rate.

In 2017, scientific studies began reporting on FMT as an experimental treatment for mental health disorders. Since it's so important for you to have as much diversity as possible in your own microbiome, the thought was that this kind of treatment might work better than probiotics, which focus on only a few strains of bacteria. FMT gives you the whole zoo!

What have the scientists found? As with all research, it tends to start with case studies, such as the successful FMT treatment of a twenty-six-year-old woman with anorexia nervosa[25] and a seventy-nine-year-old woman with treatment-resistant depression.[26] The bacterial diversity significantly increased for both at the same time as their mental health improved. A more carefully designed study was then done, with eighteen children with ASD. They were followed over eight weeks and then two years later, to see if there were short-term as well as long-term benefits of FMT.[27] Not only did these children see an improvement in their gastrointestinal symptoms, but there was also substantial benefit for ASD symptoms, with over 40 percent having minimal to no symptoms at the two-year follow-up. This was an amazing result, and hopefully more studies will be able to repeat these findings, with positive implications for ASD treatments in the future.

Another FMT study that tracked the psychological symptoms of seventeen adult patients with digestive symptoms found that 50 percent of those with depression, and 60 percent of those with anxiety, went into remission following FMT.[28] It was also found that the more depressed and anxious you were, the lower the bacterial diversity. We find these observations stunning, as they open up a whole new field of research and treatment choices for people struggling with these debilitating problems.

There are many studies underway, especially to see if the beneficial effects can be sustained over the long term. In the meantime, please don't try this at home!

Can Supplements Change the Microbiome?

Julia's research group published the first investigation into whether a broad-spectrum micronutrient formula (DEN) could change the bacteria in the microbiome of seventeen children with ADHD.[29] Ten children received multinutrients and seven received a placebo for ten weeks. The preliminary results suggested increased diversity and changes in the types of bacteria in the microbiome of the multinutrient group, which appeared to be a signal of improved microbiome health. In addition, the abundance of the genus *Bifidobacterium* in the multinutrient group dropped while it didn't in the placebo group; the more it decreased, the more the ADHD symptom scores improved. If overabundance of *Bifodobacterium* is contributing to the symptoms of ADHD, this would be a good thing to know.

Still, evaluating the microbiome over a short period of time with a small sample of children is challenging. Every person has a uniquely diverse microbiome, so it's very difficult to explore treatment-induced changes, and also to know whether the changes are meaningful and applicable to millions of people over long periods of time.

These novel results do, however, provide a basis for future research on the biological connection among ADHD, diet, and the microbiome. Previous research from Julia's lab has shown that multinutrients exert some positive effects on ADHD and associated symptoms (which you can read about in chapter 5). Taken together, the research suggests that multinutrient treatment may result in a more diverse microbiome, which may, in turn, have a positive effect on brain health.

One good thing that's come about thanks to all the research and attention now being paid to the gut microbiome is that we now know for certain how important it is for human health. Maybe instead of saying "We are what we eat," we should start saying "We are what we *absorb*." Or, as other researchers have suggested, perhaps Hippocrates' famous quote "Let food be thy medicine" should be updated to "Let food for thy microbes be thy brain medicine!"[30]

The Microbiome of the Soil: Why the Mineral Density of Soil Is So Important— and What Is Happening to It

Soil Is Not Just Dirt

We all know what dirt is: it's the dust on your desk, the stuff on your shirt that makes you wash it, and the gunk you get under your fingernails and on your shoes. Some people refer to dirt as soil that is out of place, and most of them refer to dirt as basically dead material that's really annoying when it has to be cleaned up.

But anyone who's ever spent time working on a farm or in a garden knows that *soil is not just dirt*. And it's *not* dead either; it's very much alive!

Our planet is basically a very large rock with very big puddles that we call the oceans. Over the course of the 4.5 billion years of our planet's existence, the surface of our large rock has been formed by incoming meteors and asteroids from space, magma spewed from the inner core of volcanoes, and water and wind erosion. The result is soil, the top layer of our planet's continents. It's composed of ancient minerals, water, and microbes, and the thin layer you step on is made up of fine particles that we call topsoil. Topsoil is generally only five to ten inches deep.

When you think about it, that ten inches is absolutely miniscule in relation to the 4,000-mile depth of the earth. Along with ocean life, this thin "skin" is what we depend on for our food. In other words, all of life depends upon the abundance grown from this ten-inch layer of soil with its minerals, water, and microbes.

Plants Can Synthesize Vitamins, but Humans Basically Cannot

When plants grow in healthy, well-balanced soil, they can select and use any of the 118 elements in the periodic table that they need at any point in time. Research over the years has defined fifteen as being required for plants to grow; in reality, many more may be needed, but the research on them is still incomplete. Why are those fifteen "essential" minerals so important? In part, because plants use them to synthesize approximately fifteen vitamins. We then eat the plants — or eat the animals that have eaten the plants — and that's how we get nearly all of the thirty minerals and vitamins that are currently known to be essential for our health.

People can synthesize a small amount of a few vitamins, such as vitamin K and some B vitamins, but it's not actually your human cells that are doing this. Your bacteria are! Vitamin synthesis is one of the important functions of a healthy, diverse intestinal microbiome. So even for the vitamins that we produce, we're still dependent on other organisms for this to happen. (The primary exception is vitamin D; our human skin cells pro-

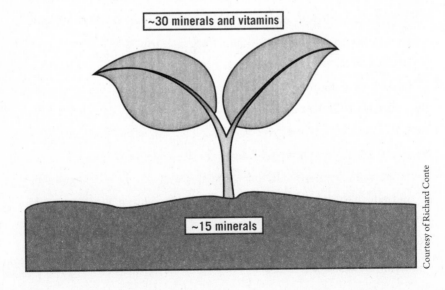

Courtesy of Richard Conte

duce it when they're exposed to sufficient sunlight.) What about all the other vitamins we need? We can *only* get them from our food or supplements.

But if some of these minerals are deficient or absent from the soil, the plants will be deficient, and then the animals or people eating the plants will be deficient.

And that is a very big problem.

Soil Microbes

If you read *The Secret Life of Trees* by Peter Wohlleben, or a similar book about plant communication, you probably never looked at trees the same way again. You would have learned about the importance of trees living in groups (forests), how trees are often biologically related and take care of each other by sharing food, and how they communicate with each other about weather, insect attacks, and other disturbances in the environment. Underground, within the soil, it is the microbes — especially fungi — that provide the network for all this to happen, a network so extensive that Wohlleben called it "the wood-wide web."

So how does this relate to brain health? Well, the fungi provide nutrients to the trees and other plants, sometimes carrying the nutrients and water across large distances. What do they get out of this? It is a beautiful example of symbiosis: the fungi feed the trees, and the trees feed the fungi. The trees use the nutrients to grow, enabling them to carry out photosynthesis in their leaves, which results in food that the trees can pass back down to the soil fungi. All of this is going on under our feet and

These microorganisms are so numerous it's estimated that there are more of them living in a teaspoon of healthy soil than there are people living on earth. It sounds very crowded! But that's what the phrase "the living soil" actually means.

around the world, because of this enormously well-developed synergy between soil microbes and plants.

Similarly, humans have a symbiotic relationship with all the microbes in our bodies.

Although fungi are particularly important for trees, they are not the only microbes living in the soil. Soil microorganisms consist primarily of bacteria, fungi, protozoa, and nematodes.

Unfortunately, just as humans have become efficient destroyers of the bacteria in human microbiomes, we have also become quite excellent at killing soil microbes.

Soil Minerals

The peach you just ate is not the same as the peach your grandmother ate. It might be as pretty, but unfortunately it is probably not as *nutritious,* and also not as *delicious.*

Are you surprised? You shouldn't be. Many things contribute to the flavor of our food, including the mineral content of our soil.

Are Nutrients in Our Food Decreasing?

Various reports have suggested that our food supply has become nutrient-poor, especially over the last seventy years. In a 2008 book by nutritionist Martina Watts, *Nutrition and Mental Health: A Handbook,* the chapter written by Dr. David Thomas and entitled "Mental Health and Mineral Depletion" summarized studies on soil mineral changes since 1940: "Collectively, there has been an average 19 percent loss in magnesium, a 29 percent loss in calcium, a 37 percent loss in iron and a really alarming 62 percent loss in copper — iron and copper being the only trace elements analyzed in 1940."

Evaluating the nutrient content of different foods over long periods of time is extremely challenging because there are so many variables. Crops have a range of varieties (you cannot say an apple is an apple is an apple!); samples are sometimes stored differently; and modern agriculture has increased the yield for so many crops that a "dilution effect" can lower nutrient levels.[31] So it's easy to criticize some of the studies, and dismiss concerns, because many changes are still within the range of natural variation.

The growing community of mostly American agricultural experts who are part of the Regenerative Agriculture movement are, fortunately, trying to do something about our current soil problems. There are now many organizations focused on improving our food supply, such as the Soil Health Academy Schools (soilhealthacademy.org), Acres USA (acresusa.com), Rodale Institute (rodaleinstitute.org), and Savory Institute (savory.global). Listen to any of their podcasts or attend any of their workshops and you will hear about the importance of soil organisms for soil health, organic and sustainable farming techniques, and holistic management of grasslands.

We just can't get complacent about whether or not there's a significant downward trend of the nutrients in our soil and crops. Instead, we should be looking at all the reasons why nutrient content is at risk right now.

What Could Cause Decreased Nutrient Density?

Farmers all know that many years of tilling the soil, even with rotating crops, depletes many minerals. That's why they use fertilizers! But most fertilizers contain only the three nutrients many of us put on our front lawn: N, P, K, which stands for nitrogen, phosphorus, and potassium. What about the rest of the minerals we need? Plants can't make them — they have to absorb them from the soil. And people can't make them either.

Some farmers add a few other minerals, such as calcium, zinc, or selenium, to their NPK fertilizer. But a lot of them don't, and some think they cannot afford them. On the other hand, one Canadian food pro-

Sick soil means sick plants, sick animals, and sick people. . . It is neither a complicated nor expensive undertaking to restore our soils to balance and thereby work a real miracle in the control of disease . . . [and] it's a moneymaking move for the farmer. . . It is simpler to cure sick soils than sick people—which will we choose?

—Dr. Charles Northen, 1936, US Congressional Record

ducer recently showed us his calculations indicating there would be *more* money in his pocket if he improved the mineral balance in his soil used to grow cereal grains. How? Because the $600 cost per acre of rebalancing could be spread over twenty years, but the improved soil and increased yield was expected to bring in much more than that.

In 2018 Bonnie was able to analyze fourteen minerals in a random sample of forty soil assays taken from fields across the four western Canadian provinces. That's a lot of acres — 30 percent of Canada's arable land! The testing looked at the recommended ranges for calcium, magnesium, potassium, sodium, boron, iron, manganese, copper, zinc, cobalt, nitrogen, sulfur, and phosphate. The results were shocking. In 98 percent of the fields, magnesium was the only mineral that consistently met the lowest acceptable level of expectations; it was followed by iron, which met the lowest level in 52 percent of the samples. The other twelve minerals all fell below acceptable levels in the majority of the samples.

Another surprising result also emerged. Bonnie was given assays from two almost adjacent fields, one organic and one not — but there was *no* difference between the two in terms of the fourteen minerals. Everyone was surprised, because we tend to think of organic farmers as being better stewards of the soil, and they probably are. But even they can be victims of poor soil quality.

If the minerals aren't in the soil, we have an enormous problem — one that isn't solved by eating organically. Organic should mean pesticide- and herbicide-free, which is a good thing, but it has nothing to do with mineral density in the soil or the nutrient density of our food.

Other Factors That May Be Compromising the Nutrient Content of Our Food

The loss of nutrients in our veggies, fruits, and grains isn't due solely to nutrient depletion in the soil. It's due to the food industry's insistence on crops that grow more quickly, and the public's demand for foods that look better instead of tasting better. Or that have a longer shelf life.

If crops are modified so that they grow more quickly, obviously they will spend less time in the soil. Will that shorter growing period allow them to absorb sufficient minerals to synthesize vitamins? Are hydroponics companies adding a full range of minerals to the water in which the plants are grown? When crops are genetically modified to be sweeter, or to ripen more quickly, or to meet any of the dozens of needs of large farms, will the higher carbohydrate content that sweetens those crops replace any of the minerals and vitamins that humans need more than sugar?

We don't have the answers to these specific questions, but we will keep asking them. Especially since we believe that human health needs are more important than convenience and consumer appeal. When it comes to genetically modified food, however, there already are a lot of answers. And the answers are very worrisome.

About Glyphosate

Glyphosate is a chemical initially patented in the United States in 1964 as a descaling agent to get rid of mineral deposits in pipes and boilers. (If you have a coffeemaker or kettle, you know how limescale can build up over time.) In the 1970s, glyphosate became the active ingredient in Roundup™, the most widely used herbicide in the world, made by Monsanto, which is now owned by Bayer. Roundup™ and glyphosate-based herbicides (GBHs) are nonselective, meaning they are designed to kill any living plant. An estimated 95 percent of the cropland in North America has been treated with Roundup™ or GBHs, even though Roundup™ has been or will be (in the not-too-distant future) banned in many countries around the world.

Is Roundup™ unhealthy for humans? It is surprisingly difficult to answer that question. Our governments seem to make decisions about chemical safety based only on whether or not these chemicals can cause cancer, and there is a lot of controversy about whether glyphosate exposure increases your cancer risk. The first major court case supported the plaintiffs who sued Monsanto because of their affliction with cancer, and their final adjusted settlement in August 2018 was $80 million. There are over 85,000 Roundup™ cancer lawsuits still pending.

It's also impossible to talk about glyphosate without talking about genetically modified (GM) crops, which were first released to food producers in the United States in 1996. Why? Because the primary purpose of the majority of those genetic modifications is to enable crops to survive when a field is treated with glyphosate. In other words, the GM seeds are resistant to herbicides as well as to some insects that are targeted. They are usually called Roundup Ready® seeds.

Despite a lot of conflicting research on glyphosate and cancer, there is even less knowledge about its impact on other areas of health, although glyphosate and other herbicides have an obviously detrimental impact on the environment, affecting animals and other plants as excess levels remain in the area or are washed into watersheds. In particular, very few scientists have been studying glyphosate's impact on the brain. That may change now that a 2019 study showed that glyphosate disturbs the human blood-brain barrier, making it more permeable.[32] This means that some molecules that the blood-brain barrier is intended to exclude might be passing through and causing adverse effects in our brains.

Another problem with glyphosate involves timing. Glyphosate was thought to be safe by many farmers who use it only in the early stage of plant growth, because they believed it washed away over time as the plants grew bigger. But now many countries, including the United States and Canada, have approved glyphosate as a desiccant — a pre-harvest aid, or drying agent. When is a desiccant applied to crops? Five to ten days before the harvest, if the fields are weed-infested or the grain moisture content is too high for efficient harvesting. As a result, some studies have shown that there is residual glyphosate in many types of flours and cereals, probably because of its application so late in the growth cycle.[33]

Is the amount being detected in our food supply safe? No one knows for sure, certainly not in terms of brain health. But the small amount of research we have found on the impact of glyphosate on nutrient quality of plants is very concerning. That's because glyphosate makes the dietary minerals like iron, manganese, and nickel *less* available for your body to absorb.[34] This is hardly surprising, because glyphosate's first job when initially patented was to *remove* minerals!

There is another important economic consideration. Plants grown in healthy, balanced soil are more resistant to insects, reducing the need for pesticides. It costs money for a farmer to balance the soil by adding minerals, and it can take two to four years to complete the task. So unbalanced soil creates a huge market for herbicides, fungicides, and pesticides, which the chemical companies are happy to sell.

One of the biggest challenges in the glyphosate situation is that there are no universally accepted standards to compensate food producers for quality. Quantity, yes; the economic incentive is to focus on the volume of the harvest.

Finally, we note that even though we specified glyphosate in the discussion above, much of what we are saying applies to other — and future — chemicals. Companies such as Bayer have developed new chemicals to replace glyphosate because weeds have developed a resistance to it. The new chemicals are being released now and many more are anticipated by 2030. This new development is unlikely to be good news. If only they focused instead on returning the soil to its natural, mineralized state — healthy soil leads to healthy plants that are pest-resistant on their own.

Glyphosate and Your Intestinal Microbiome

In 2019, it was proven that one way glyphosate kills plants is by interfering with a biochemical pathway (called the shikimate pathway) that is important for the production of the aromatic amino acids, some of the building blocks of proteins.[35] Many strains of the bacteria found in the human gut microbiome also have this pathway — which raises an inevitable question. Are human health problems in the gastrointestinal system being triggered by glyphosate?

Various studies have found that glyphosate was associated with changes in animal microbiomes, as well as lesions associated with fatty liver disease.[36] There are a lot of studies showing that GM crops do not seem to affect the health of some animals, mainly birds and fish, or mammals that are physiologically different from humans. But recently an extensive investigation was done in pigs, which, of all animals, are metabolically the most similar to humans. (This is the reason substances related to metabolic pathways are first tested in pigs before being tested in people.) Thus it is particularly relevant that this study of GM soy and maize showed that 32 percent of the GM-fed pigs had severe stomach inflammation, and it was four times worse in males than females.[37]

Many experts suggest that when people have difficulty digesting some types of food, especially wheat gluten and dairy, their intestinal reactions may actually be caused by residual glyphosate, not by the gluten or milk protein.[38] We are so saturated by glyphosate in our food now that it is very hard to find the true cause. And we know that glyphosate residue can attack our beneficial gut bugs and harm the protective lining of our digestive tracts.[39]

Last but not least, glyphosate is a patented antibiotic that interrupts microbiome pathways and harms certain bacteria. (Yes, bacteria have microbiomes too!) Glyphosate adversely affects the balance of microorganisms in the soil. It reduces the population of beneficial organisms and increases the population of opportunistic organisms. The soil no longer acts vibrant and alive. It looks more like the dead substance we call dirt.

What can the individual do? A carefully controlled study of urinary glyphosate (and its main metabolite) in sixteen adults and children who did not normally eat organic food was recently reported.[40] Over the course of six days, everyone followed an organic diet and submitted urine samples to the scientists. The result was a 70 percent drop in glyphosate and its main metabolite by the end of the week for all participants. Eating organic food can be expensive, but this is evidence that it does reduce our body burden of this chemical.

Climate Change

Another cause of crop nutrient deficiency may be higher levels of carbon dioxide in the atmosphere. In fact, recent estimates are that climate change may rob our diet of much of the iron, zinc, and protein that we need, unless these nutrients are supplemented in the soil or our food.[41]

This is a paradox! Plants *like* carbon and they use it to grow more. But the problem is that more carbon dioxide also leads to plants containing fewer micronutrients and more sugars; the plants are bigger and much of the food tastes sweeter, but it's not giving us more micronutrients for brain health. Some people say it's just creating sugar bombs: produce with lots of carbohydrates to fill us up, but not much nutrition to help our brains function.

One study looked at nutrient balance in spring wheat grown for three consecutive seasons.[42] Higher carbon dioxide levels led to larger plants and a higher yield, but there was more than a 7 percent decline in protein, a significant decrease in iron and manganese, and an increase in carbohydrates. Similar results have been found in studies of other grains and cereals.

Overall, it appears that our plants will become higher in carbohydrates and lower in protein and micronutrients as our planet heats up. More research is needed on these very important issues because of their impact on human health.

Studies on Mineral Deficiencies and Mental Health

In 1991 Dr. Melvyn Werbach at UCLA published a sourcebook entitled *Nutritional Influences on Mental Illness.* In it, he reviewed all the literature up to that time on nutrients that were shown to affect everything from A (aggressive behavior, anxiety, ADHD, anxiety) to S (schizophrenia). Then, in *Nutrition and Mental Health: A Handbook,* published in 2008, the results of 214 peer-reviewed research papers from 1940 to 2002 that related mental disorders to mineral deficiencies or imbalances were summarized by Dr. David Thomas as follows:

- ADHD has been correlated with deficiencies in copper, magnesium, phosphorous, and zinc
- Anxiety has been correlated with deficiencies in potassium, magnesium, phosphorus, and selenium
- Aggression has been correlated with deficiencies in iron, potassium, and zinc
- Bipolar disorder has been correlated with deficiencies in iron, iodine, potassium, magnesium, molybdenum, and vanadium
- Depression has been correlated with deficiencies of almost every mineral evaluated, with the exceptions of molybdenum and phosphorus

- PMS has been correlated with deficiencies in copper, iron, magnesium, and zinc
- Schizophrenia has been correlated with deficiencies in copper, iron, iodine, magnesium, and selenium

There are two noteworthy conclusions to be drawn from this information. First, as we discuss in the next chapter, correlations do not provide proof of causation. However, the information above does reveal a strong pattern of mineral deficiencies across all mental health problems evaluated, and the information is derived from studies across sixty years. And second, the information demonstrates the fallacy of the magic bullet thinking described in the Introduction.

How Consumer Demand Can Influence Nutrient Density

As a consumer, you have the power to influence the nutrient density of your food!

- *Seasonal eating* is a good place to start. Fresh produce is more nutritious than produce that has been stored for weeks. What's left when the nutrients decline? Carbohydrates — which are converted to sugar in your body and stored as fat . . . which leads to weight gain. Even though this can be a challenge for those of us living in colder climates, choose local, freshly picked produce whenever you can. If you buy it at a farmer's market, you can also discuss growing methods, potential use of herbicides like glyphosate, and soil condition with the farmers themselves.
- We know of companies developing apps and handheld devices that will enable consumers to evaluate the nutrient content of fresh pro-

duce in the grocery store before buying it. Watch for these to come onto the market, and when they do, grab them and *use* them! We'll be able to show grocery stores that we care about more than our food's appearance: we care about nutrient density. (The success of Imperfect Foods, a home delivery service that is spreading across the United States, dedicated to reducing food waste by providing good produce that is misshapen or ugly, is proof that people care about quality over appearance.)

- Be aware of how your food is grown, and where. An educated public that demands nutrient-dense food with no herbicide or pesticide residue will eventually see changes. A decade or two ago, who would have imagined that there would be so many organic and plant-based foods for sale now in local supermarkets?

- The Environmental Working Group's website (ewg.org) is an excellent resource for information about ongoing struggles with this issue.

- American certified crop adviser Jim Porterfield offers this succinct summary: "Eat fresh, certified organic vegetables grown locally in minerally balanced soil." He points out that there are about four million acres of vegetables and fruit in the United States. Even if it took $4,000 per acre to detoxify those soils and balance the soil minerals to grow vegetables, that would be equivalent to the cost of about sixteen Stealth bombers. What a change could be made in soil and human health in one growing season!

Mother Nature has neatly packaged nutrients together that are needed together. But to rely on Mother Nature, we need to return to healthy farming practices.

The Takeaway

1. Microbes inhabit many parts of your body, especially the gastrointestinal tract. Feeding your microbes with prebiotics (the nondigestible fiber found in many plant-based foods) will enable these tiny organisms to function at their best, which is important for our own health.

2. The health and diversity of your unique intestinal microbiome may be affecting your mental health, although the evidence base is not strong so far. As often happens, the hype has exceeded the scientific data, and there are many claims made for probiotic treatment of mental health challenges.

3. Another important microbiome is in our soil. The importance of dietary minerals is underestimated by the public. Most people don't realize that without adequate minerals in the soil, plants can't produce the vitamins we need. Depletion of soil minerals jeopardizes our ability to get the nutrients we need even if we eat a super-healthy diet.

4. The overuse of herbicides like glyphosate and other chemicals has had a severe impact on how crops are grown as well as their nutritional value, and we don't know how much of these chemicals we're absorbing every time we eat.

5. Climate change is also likely lowering micronutrient levels in food while increasing carbohydrate levels.

Part II

BETTER NUTRITION
FOR A BETTER BRAIN

4

THE POWER OF THE FOOD YOU EAT

FOR THOSE OF US who study mental health and nutrition, the last decade has been incredibly exciting, with so much research coming together to show how the nutrients we consume influence how we feel, sleep, concentrate, and cope with stress. So in this part of the book, we are sharing the very best of this research — and we've been particularly mindful not to cherry-pick studies that show nutrients only in a positive light. We want you to see how amazingly potent the results of these studies are.

This research proves the point of this book, including addressing an important question about the direction of causality: Which comes first? Does eating a mostly processed diet *cause* anxiety and depression? Or . . . are people who are anxious and depressed just more likely to crave processed foods? Is that, in fact, why we call some of them comfort foods? As we often say, a depressed person rarely craves broccoli — so can we prove that a mostly processed diet is causing depression and not vice versa?

First, we will show you that what we eat correlates with our mental health. But then, in order to determine the direction of causality, we will look at prospective studies that ask whether the nutrient-poor diet *precedes* the onset of mental health problems (it does), and then whether improving your diet results in improved mental health (and it does). Then in the next few chapters we'll cover the last step: determining whether adding the right types of nutrient supplements improves mental health (and it does!).

Let's take a look at some of the most illuminating studies.

Do the Eating Habits of Population Groups Correlate with Their Mental Health?

In a cross-sectional, correlational study, all the variables are measured at the same time point and examined for relationships. For example, a researcher might ask people if they have any symptoms of depression, and also what they tend to eat.

The connections revealed in correlational studies can be completely random. Tyler Vigen's book *Spurious Correlations* cleverly illustrates this. He showed that people who eat cheese are more likely to die by becoming tangled in their bedsheets than those who don't eat cheese (maybe cheese affects sleep?), and the divorce rate in Maine is beautifully correlated with eating margarine (maybe margarine makes you more irritable?). The point is that we can never draw conclusions about causation from correlational studies.

Even though correlational studies are often considered weak because they can't prove causation, sometimes there are many studies using pretty much identical methods across many different cultures that generate pretty much identical findings. When that happens, then the sheer weight of that evidence can be very influential. So what we want to focus on now is an example of that. There have been more than a dozen studies from all over the world, *categorizing* dietary patterns and *correlating* those patterns with some type of mental health problem. It doesn't matter whether they refer to their comparisons as healthy vs. unhealthy diets, whole or true foods vs. processed food, Mediterranean vs. Western diets — the common denominator is a comparison of real food to processed nutrient-poor food.

What have they all found? Food seems to matter. A lot.

For example, a study of over a thousand Australian women showed that a "traditional" dietary pattern of vegetables, fruit, meat, fish, and whole grains was associated with *lower* odds for depression and anxiety disorders.[1] They also showed

No matter how old you are, if you eat healthier whole foods, you're more likely to have lower scores on depression and anxiety scales than if you eat a more processed diet.

that a Western diet of processed or fried foods, refined grains, sugary products, and beer was associated with *more* mental health symptoms.

Other studies have focused on the role of diet in relation to ADHD symptoms. One from Korea that looked at almost 17,000 children noted that ADHD symptoms were correlated with a higher consumption of unhealthy items like fast food, soft drinks, and instant noodles and not with higher consumption of fruit and vegetables.[2]

Some studies have explored what *form* you consume your fruit and vegetables in — raw, canned, or cooked. A New Zealand study found that *raw* fruit and vegetable intake was more strongly associated with improved wellness as compared to canned or cooked fruit and vegetables.[3] The top ten raw foods related to better mental health were carrots, bananas, apples, dark leafy greens like spinach, grapefruit, lettuce, citrus fruits, fresh berries, cucumber, and kiwifruit. This might be due to the fact that raw foods contain more minerals and vitamins, as the heat of cooking can destroy some vitamins. In fact, the longer you cook a food, the more the heat destroys the vitamins (that's why some people like microwaving — it's fast!).

The Canadian Community Health Survey collects nationwide information across Canada. In a CCHS study on the economic burden of poor eating habits, 80 percent of the women and 89 percent of the men were eating fewer servings of fruits and veggies than recommended by Health

Canada (five to nine half-cup servings per day) — a rate that is typical for much of the Western world. But what these researchers highlighted was the healthcare cost of *not* eating these foods — it was determined to be 3.3 billion Canadian dollars per year![4]

What's astonishing about these data is that over the next twenty years, an increase of *just one serving of vegetables and fruit per day* would save approximately 9.2 billion Canadian dollars in healthcare costs. In a country like Canada, with one-tenth the population of the United States, that is an amazing number.

How does the United States compare? The National Health and Nutrition Examination Survey showed that over 30 percent of the average adult caloric intake is from low-nutrient-density foods, and that consumption of these processed foods was associated with low intake of dietary nutrients overall.[5] A University of North Carolina study of over 150,000 American households reported that more than three-quarters of the energy in products purchased by Americans from 2000 to 2012 came from moderately and highly processed foods.[6] That is very sobering information about the prevalence of processed food in the typical American diet. Results contained in a recent CDC report were even more dramatic: in 2015 only about 9 percent of Americans were eating the recommended number of daily vegetable servings.[7] Canada's data are similar: an analysis of the 2004 CCHS data reported that 48 percent of the caloric intake across Canada came from nutrient-poor ultra-processed foods.[8]

And how do these eating patterns relate to *mental* health? In 2017, Bonnie and her colleague Dr. Karen Davison analyzed data looking at food insecurity, diet quality, and perceived mental health in more than 15,000 adults aged nineteen to seventy years.[9] They found that both food insecurity and poor diet quality were correlated with a 60 percent increased probability of reporting poor mental health.

Fish Consumption and Mental Symptoms

Many epidemiological studies also show that it's time to go fishing. Or at least go to your local fishmonger for some lovely salmon or mackerel for your dinner.

We've known for a long time that countries where the population eats a lot of fish have a lowered rate of a whole host of psychiatric problems. In fact, low seafood consumption is associated with a sixty-five-times higher lifetime risk for depression, a fifty times higher risk for postpartum depression, and a thirty times higher risk for bipolar disorder.[10]

These numbers are extraordinary! And there are likely other reasons for these huge effects, such as socioeconomic status, or that people who don't eat fish also don't eat other foods that are good for the brain.

What conclusion can be drawn from all these correlational data? *People who eat a healthier diet have fewer mental health problems.*

Do Dietary Habits *Predict* the Onset of Mental Health Problems?

Thanks to several studies published in the last decade, we now know that poor diet seems to *precede* poor mental health. A whole food diet, on the other hand, is *protective.*

A prospective study in the United Kingdom looked at more than 3,000 middle-aged people whose dietary pattern mainly consisted of sweet desserts, fried food, processed meat, and refined grains.[11] Their diet was a risk factor for the emergence of depression five years later — but eating whole foods like vegetables, fruit, and fish was protective. This study was soon followed by an even larger one of over 9,000 adults in Spain who were not depressed or taking antidepressants. Everyone in this SUN project (mentioned in chapter 2) provided information about their regular dietary intake, and Dr. Almudena Sanchez-Villegas and her colleagues watched for new cases of depression to develop.[12] Almost 500 new cases of depression had emerged at the six-year mark, and a higher risk of depression was related to consumption of fast food and commercially baked goods.

A Canadian study evaluated more than 3,000 children aged ten and eleven for the number of good health behaviors they were practicing — mostly related to diet, but some on exercise and daily screen time.[13] Then the scientists waited two years before looking at government data indicating which children were referred to a physician for treatment of a mental health disorder. Not only did children who followed more of the good health behaviors remain more mentally healthy, but for every single additional health guideline children adhered to, there were 15 percent fewer visits for medical treatment of mental health problems. Further analyses showed that meeting recommendations for fruit and vegetable, meat, saturated fat, and sugar consumption was associated with fewer ADHD diagnoses.[14] Think of the cost savings and enhanced health outcomes if dietary intake were improved across the whole population!

More and more reports are coming in about young people, including one that evaluated the diets of more than 3,000 adolescents in Australia.[15] Not surprisingly, the highest intake of unhealthy foods was correlated with poorer mental health functioning, while the highest intake of healthy foods was associated with better mental health functioning. The progression over time was even more interesting: those who improved their diet over two years also improved their mental health, while those whose diet got worse had poorer psychological functioning. Given that adolescence is a time when it's harder for parents to supervise their children's diet — as well as a time of great vulnerability to developing mental health problems — the results of this study are extremely important. The good news is that we will show you it's incredibly easy to change your diet and improve your mental health at the same time.

However, not all studies show these associations. For example, a study of almost 4,000 adolescents did not find that fruit and vegetable consumption was associated with the development of depression twelve years later, showing that prediction of these disorders over a long period of time is challenging and multifactorial.[16]

Finally, a remarkable study about suicide in Japan followed close to 100,000 people for four years.[17] They found that a dietary pattern with a high consumption of vegetables, fruits, mushrooms, seaweed, and fish was related to about a 50 percent *decreased* risk of death from suicide four years later. Given that suicide is an escalating problem all over the world, this study is certainly one we should pay attention to. What is most noteworthy about all these data? *Not one study has shown that the Western diet is good for our mental health.*

Pregnancy, Diet, and Mental Health

Many women are thrilled to be pregnant, while others can feel much more vulnerable as they worry about the onset or relapse of mental health problems.

The most common mental health problems during pregnancy are anxiety and depression, which are among the leading causes of maternal illness and mortality worldwide.[18] Research shows that the poorer the diet quality, the greater the likelihood of depressive and stress symptoms during the prenatal period as well as immediately after the baby's birth. Also, the healthier the diet, the lower the rate of these symptoms.[19]

But what about the offspring? How does a pregnant mom's diet affect them?

We've known for decades that severe malnutrition during pregnancy can lead to mental health problems in the offspring. Two large-scale famines taught us the importance of prenatal nutrition: the Dutch Hunger Winter of 1944–45 and a severe famine in China in 1959–61 showed that women malnourished in pregnancy had over twice the risk of producing offspring who went on to develop schizophrenia and depression.[20]

These are extreme examples, but we do now know that eating fewer nourishing foods during pregnancy is not helpful for the baby. While women are likely to know that they should avoid raw fish, raw eggs, and unwashed produce during pregnancy, they may not know the role that low-nutrient ultra-processed foods are playing in their child's development.

A study based on more than 23,000 Norwegian mother-child pairs showed that mothers who ate more processed food during pregnancy were more likely to have children with behavioral problems five years later.[21] A French study, with about 1,200 mother-child pairs, showed that a typical Western diet during pregnancy increased the chances of the child displaying hyperactivity and inattention at ages three, five, and eight years.[22] A Dutch study of more than 3,000 pregnant women showed that the traditional Dutch Diet, with lots of fresh and processed meat and potatoes, a relatively high intake of margarine, and a very low intake of eggs, vegetables, fish, and dairy products, was associated with more aggression in their offspring at age six.[23] In contrast, a study of about 700 mother-infant pairs in Norway showed that increased fruit consumption during pregnancy was associated with enhanced cognitive development of the infant at one year.[24]

Many women who were worried about too much mercury in their fish stopped eating any, but a low intake of omega-3s during pregnancy is a greater risk for her offspring than the small amount of exposure to mercury. The current scientific advice is that eating fish in pregnancy is good for both mother and child,[25] and the general recommendation is to eat fish once or twice a week. On the other hand, as we have known for many years, it is wise for all of us to avoid obtaining too high a proportion of our fish intake from the larger fish (e.g., swordfish, tuna), as they tend to have a higher concentration of mercury.

If People Learn How to Change Their Eating Habits, Does Their Mental Health Improve?

What happens if we can convince people to change their diet? The first well-crafted studies investigating diet change and mental health came about thanks to a pediatric allergist named Dr. Benjamin Feingold, who published in 1975 a very popular book called *Why Your Child Is Hyperactive*. Many thousands of families of children with ADHD have followed the Feingold diet, because he saw hyperactive, impulsive, and inattentive symptoms improve in his young patients when artificial colors, salicylates, and petroleum-based preservatives were removed from their diets. But even though many families insisted that the Feingold diet vastly improved their children's behavior, initial studies of the diet's effectiveness were mixed.[26]

Further studies, including one of Bonnie's first RCTs (randomized controlled trials) in children with ADHD,[27] showed that eating less processed and additive-laden food helped with ADHD symptoms. (A randomized controlled trial is one that is highly controlled, often very selective about participants, and usually involves the use of some kind of placebo or another established intervention as a comparator.) Other studies continued to appear, confirming what Dr. Feingold knew: food preservatives and artificial colors can affect the behavior of some children. Overall, it appears that about one-third of ADHD children respond to a dietary intervention that eliminates possible culprits like artificial colors and preservatives, as well as other possible food allergens.[28] However, when stimulant meds became widely prescribed for ADHD in the 1980s and 1990s, the public (and scientists) largely lost interest in the role of diet.

In 2012, Dr. Joel Nigg, professor of psychology at Oregon Health & Science University, reviewed this literature and concluded that the effect of just food dyes alone, while small, showed that about 8 percent of children could benefit from their elimination.[29] This might seem like a tiny number — but it's not! In the United States, more than 5 *million* children are medicated for ADHD, and the numbers are growing. Eight percent represents several hundred thousand children who might have their symptoms completely eliminated if food colors were removed from their diet. Don't you think those parents would want to know about this choice? And given that the number of additives and colors has increased — consumption of food dyes increased sixfold from 1950 to 2010 — the impact of these dyes has likely increased as well. We need to consider why these substances aren't more restricted when they have zero nutritional value yet may harm an awful lot of people.

Most European companies have reformulated their products to exclude food dyes, as they have no health benefits. A new law stipulated that red dye 40 and two yellow dyes could be used only if a warning was placed on the label that these could cause "an adverse effect on activity and attention in children." But in the United States, the FDA has not mandated any such warnings. Many American food businesses and restaurants have voluntarily eliminated dyes or pledged to do so — they know it's smart business for educated consumers. In addition, at the end of 2018, the FDA announced they would remove approval of seven synthetic flavoring agents (the names of which most of us would not even recognize) — not because of negative effects on children's behavior, but because research in lab animals had shown an association with cancer.

After forty years of studies on food additives, no one can yet answer this question: How much of the children's behavior improvement is due to removal of food additives, and how much is due to the higher intake of minerals and vitamins in the food that replaced those chemicals?

While these studies do not suggest that healthier diets are a magic bullet for all children with psychological challenges, there appears to be a subgroup of children who improve dramatically on restricted diets. For them, the impact can be life-changing. These chemicals should not be allowed into our food supply until proven to be universally safe, especially as they're only used to make food look better, not *be* better.

When People Learn How to Eat a Healthier Diet, Their Symptoms of Depression Decrease

One recent study asked a simple question. In adults with depression who eat a poor diet, does teaching them about nutrition have an impact on their mental health? After the study, the answer was yes.

This study, called SMILES (Supporting the Modification of Lifestyle Interventions in Lowered Emotional States), was carried out by Professor Felice Jacka and her colleagues in Australia over twelve weeks.[30] Participants had to have previously experienced a major depressive episode, and they also had to report that they ate a typical unhealthy diet with a high intake of sweets, processed meats, and salty snacks. Then they were assigned to get either dietary support (DS) or social support (SS).

Those in the DS group had seven hours of training with a dietitian to learn about a whole foods Mediterranean diet approach (which you'll read about in Part III). Those assigned to SS received a similar amount of time in a "befriending arrangement." After the study was completed, the people who improved their diets the most were the ones who experienced the most improvement in mood. Remarkably, 32 percent of the DS group went into remission for their depression (compared to 8 percent of the SS group).

One of the incidental bits of information from this study was very important. The researchers screened 166 referrals in order to find the 67 who were randomized; in other words, 99 were screened out for various reasons. But only 15 of the 99 excluded were screened out because they had a diet that was "too good." To express it another way, only 15 out of 166 (9 percent) of a group of adults with depression met Australian guidelines for having a good diet.

One reason this study has had such a global impact was that it was followed very quickly by the HELFIMED study by Dr. Natalie Parletta (Healthy Eating for LiFe with a MEDiterranean-style diet) that had similar results.[31] And, in 2019, it was followed by a third study, targeting depressed young adults aged seventeen to thirty-five, over three weeks.[32] What was amazing about this last study, led by Dr. Heather Francis, was that the diet intervention was all done via a thirteen-minute video, with no direct contact with dietitians. This is fantastic news, as it means that people can be taught how to improve their diets no matter where they live, as long as they can get online. Other research shows that *giving* people fruit can improve their feeling of vitality, flourishing, and motivation in comparison with people who are just *told* to eat more fruit,[33] and simply adding wild blueberries can improve the mood of adolescents (12–17 years) over just four weeks.[34]

While many of these studies cannot keep their participants blind to what treatment they are receiving, the replication across different universities and geographical locations gives us confidence that these observations are robust.

How a Healthier Diet Could Influence the Treatment Gap

Alan Kazdin, a clinical psychologist and professor emeritus at Yale, has been focusing his recent research on the treatment gap.[35] This refers to the difference between the proportion of the population in need of services and the proportion that actually receive them. The numbers are staggering—because 50 percent of those with a mental health problem in the United States (approximately 35 million Americans) are not receiving *any* *help* at all for their problems. Worldwide, based on 20 percent of the population having a mental disorder in any given year, we estimate the treatment gap is close to *600 million* people. (And these numbers are from before the COVID-19 pandemic!)

Kazdin's point is that to effectively reach all of these sufferers, training more psychologists and other mental health professionals is simply not going to cut it. There are too few, the problem is too big, and training takes too long (and is very costly). And even if people are seen by a therapist, at best 50 percent of them recover.[36]

What we really need are treatments that are easy to follow and affordable. The more we can use treatments that maximize reach — like online videos or simply giving out fruit — the more people we might be able to help.

A comment from TEDx viewer Steve sums it up: "It's so funny to me that making 'healthy' food choices is stigmatized and thought of as weird, where one hundred years ago, whole, unprocessed 'healthy' food was the majority of food choices available and people were much healthier and stronger. I knew these ideas to be true when back in high school I decided to start eating 'right' and made tremendous improvements in my mental and physical health."

But . . . what if you don't get better even eating a healthy diet? Is it possible that some people might *need* more than just a change in diet? Based on what you've read already, we think you know that the answer is yes. We have both witnessed people who had incredibly good diets who continued to struggle with debilitating mood symptoms that got better only when additional nutrients were provided in pill form. The next chapter will explain why.

The Takeaway

1. Many rigorous studies have shown that there is a relationship between how people eat and how they feel. They've also shown that, often, eating poorly tends to precede poor mental health, whereas a healthy diet of whole foods is protective.

2. More than half of the food intake in North America is now drawn from the lowest level: ultra-processed "food." In other words, more than half of what we now put into our mouths has *virtually no micronutrient content.* It consists of sugars, fats, and chemicals, but not minerals and vitamins. This is a huge cause for concern and may relate to the current epidemic of mental health problems.

3. The quality of a pregnant woman's diet can affect the future mental health of her baby.

4. The good news is that excellent research now shows that being taught about healthy eating by experts—whether in person or virtually—can have a big impact on how well people eat, and also on their mental health. This type of whole-diet-treatment research can be difficult to do, but all three of the independent studies published so far have shown that education about better food choices changes the way people eat, resulting in substantial improvements in their mental health that are comparable to benefits observed with medications—and without the side effects.

5

TREATING PSYCHIATRIC DISORDERS WITH SUPPLEMENTS

IF PEOPLE WITH MENTAL health challenges consume nutrients as supplements, will this improve their mental health?

The answer to this is, often, a resounding yes.

As you've learned already, making changes in your diet is the most important first step toward better mental (and physical) health — but sometimes making excellent, healthy dietary changes just isn't enough to resolve mental health problems. You've also learned that no single nutrient works as a magic bullet solution. So in the next three chapters, we're going to review the research on *broad-spectrum* multinutrient treatments. We're going to share studies using lots of different scientific methods so that you can appreciate the weight of the evidence and make informed choices about potential treatments.

Note, however, that we often say *symptoms* instead of relying on psychiatric diagnostic categories. Why? Because we've repeatedly seen people take a broad-spectrum formula for one problem, who then are happy to report across-the-board improvements in their mental health. Often, they are sleeping better, coping with stress better, and/or feeling more energy. These unexpected reports indicate that the nutrients are having a broad effect of improving brain health.

ADHD

There has been a wealth of global research using many different types of study designs to look at the effect of broad-spectrum multinutrients on ADHD behaviors. All of the experimental designs using a broad-spectrum approach have shown substantial reduction in ADHD symptoms (based on group data) and other related behaviors. Two of the most rigorous studies were completed in Julia's lab in New Zealand.

Julia's first RCT used the broad-spectrum multinutrient supplement EMPowerplus (EMP), and followed eighty medication-free adults diagnosed with ADHD, who were randomly chosen to receive either multinutrients or a placebo for eight weeks.[1] The main outcomes were ADHD symptoms, mood, and overall functioning.

The first key finding was about the effect of the treatment. When the statistician "broke the blind" — meaning we were able to see what each participant had been taking — it was clear that the group of people who took the nutrients did better than the group who took the placebo across a number of different symptoms, including impulsivity, inattention, and overall functioning. Also, for those who entered the trial with moderate to severe depression, there was a greater improvement in mood for those who were randomized to the multinutrients as compared with those randomized to placebo. This was the first controlled trial to show that the benefit of multinutrients for the treatment of ADHD symptoms was not simply due to the placebo effect.

The second key finding was that there were minimal side effects, with no difference between groups. And all reported side effects were mild, like a headache or a bit of an upset stomach. This is great news, as many of the medications prescribed for ADHD come with side effects that some people find intolerable, such as insomnia and severe loss of appetite. The medications can be so problematic that some prefer to live with their ADHD symptoms rather than continuing to take the meds.

Four years later, one of Julia's former PhD students, Dr. Kathryn Darling, coordinated a large replication study, but this time in children with ADHD.[2] Being able to reproduce a study's results is very important in science as it helps establish the veracity of the effect being observed. What did the new study find?

In this study, ninety-three medication-free children with ADHD, aged seven to twelve, were randomly assigned to take either the broad-spectrum multinutrient supplement Daily Essential Nutrients (DEN) or placebo capsules for ten weeks. Inattention and overall functioning improved more in children who took the nutrients than in those who took the placebo. There were no group differences in hyperactivity/impulsivity.

After observing hundreds of people taking these multinutrient formulas, we believe their primary effect is on the ability to regulate emotions. Improved self-regulation leads to a more stable mood, reduced irritability and aggression, feelings of inner calm, better sleep, and, over time, better focus and clarity of thought. Many people report that they feel the fog in their brain lifting.

Across all raters (parents, teachers, and clinicians), there was greater improvement in emotion regulation and aggression for those children who took the multinutrients compared to the placebo group. One of these children was Isaiah (he asked we use his real name), one of the many success stories from this clinical trial.

How Isaiah Conquered His ADHD

Isaiah was nine when he started in one of Julia's nutrient studies. He was unable to brush his teeth or tie his shoelaces. He had been expelled from six preschools and several schools because of his ADHD and severe aggression toward other children.

Now seventeen, he is an avid and talented skateboarder and has caught up on seven years of schooling.

He and his parents credit the micronutrients for his "amazing progress."

Isaiah's mother heard about the trial and told us she had "nothing to lose." Previously, Isaiah had tried many different types of ADHD medication, but they made his anxiety worse and caused heart problems. She told us that "he became zombified enough to sit in school, but the exuberant little boy I knew was gone." Isaiah agreed. He hated how the medications made him feel. They had reached the end of the road as to what psychiatry and medication could offer them.

Isaiah was randomly chosen to be in the multinutrient group (although neither he nor the researchers knew it at the time) and within weeks his parents were noticing a substantial improvement in his behavior. Before the trial, they would get phone calls from the school every day, and Isaiah would often be sent home due to his challenging behaviors. The phone calls stopped.

After the study ended, we continued to track Isaiah's ADHD symptoms and other behaviors. He is now academically on track, calm, and motivated for his future, his severe ADHD symptoms are much better, and the most exciting result is that Isaiah is happy. His mother told us the nutrients "have absolutely saved our lives as a family."

In each of these studies, about half of the participants taking the supplement were rated as "much" to "very much improved" by the clinicians.

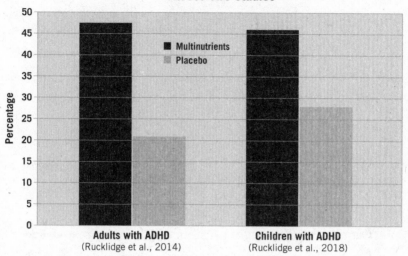

From *Journal of Child and Adolescent Psychopharmacology* 12, Issue 3, by permission of Mary Ann Liebert, Inc.

The graph illustrates the rate of response across the multinutrient and placebo conditions for both the adult and child RCTs. This means that the clinicians observed substantial and noticeable improvement across a range of symptoms, with significant benefit on overall functioning. A further 30 percent showed a milder improvement, whereas the remaining 20 percent showed no benefit. Both studies showed remarkable consistency for improved regulation of emotions.

The participants in both RCTs were followed for one year after the study began. Because people were no longer reporting how they felt in controlled circumstances, quite a bit of bias can creep in during this type of follow-up, but these studies allow us to evaluate effectiveness in real life. Happily, the results from both follow-ups were remarkably similar.[3] About 20 percent of the participants kept taking the nutrients, and they were found to be doing better than those who chose to stop taking them.

We also found continued improvement over time for those who stayed

In both RCTs with adults and children with ADHD, about 80 percent of those taking the broad-spectrum multinutrient formulas were in remission at the one-year follow-up from their ADHD symptoms compared to only 40 percent of those taking medications and 20 percent of those who were taking nothing.

on the nutrients, suggesting that the benefit of the multinutrient treatment takes time to reach its full potential. In all areas of functioning, those who stayed on the nutrients the longest were doing the best.

We also found that those who switched from nutrients to medications like Ritalin were more likely to have problems with mood or anxiety at the one-year follow-up assessment. You might be wondering why many preferred medication and stopped taking the nutrients: the primary reason was cost. There is an even larger controlled trial with ADHD kids underway (results expected by early 2021) led by one of Julia's former students, Dr. Jeni Johnstone, at Oregon Health & Science University in Portland.[4] It involves three centers (two in the United States and one in Canada).

Nutrients or Medications for ADHD?

Julia has studied the treatment of ADHD with broad-spectrum multinutrient formulas more than anyone else in the world. If you're wondering whether to choose multinutrients or medications, this is her advice:

1. If you're looking for a treatment that has a quick impact (within a few hours), multinutrients will simply not work as quickly as stimulant medication. Stimulants show much larger and more powerful changes in core ADHD symptoms in the short term. In contrast, the effects of multinutrients

are subtler, but grow over time with longer exposure. The exception is for symptoms like explosive rage; for that, we routinely see improvements in just a few days with broad-spectrum multinutrients.

2. Of course not all children respond to multinutrients—but for those who do benefit, the effects are substantial and are often seen across all areas of functioning. These effects, such as improved sleep and mood or reduced aggression, are usually not found in studies of stimulant medication.

3. The side effect profile for multinutrients is better, with no substantial effects reported on sleep or appetite, unless they are taken too close to bedtime. (B vitamins tend to energize.) We also hear anecdotally that children are healthier—skin conditions clear up, fewer colds, fewer infections—when taking additional nutrients with their diet.

4. Taking multinutrients means taking more capsules, and more often. Some families find it difficult to ensure long-term compliance with taking the nutrients three times a day.

5. There is no rebound effect associated with taking multinutrients (an effect often observed with medications as the drug wears off). Irritability tends to get better, not worse.

6. In our research, teachers did not note improvements in core ADHD symptoms such as attention whereas research with stimulant medication has repeatedly found strong effects based on teacher ratings. Teachers identified improved behavior regulation and reduced aggression in children taking the multinutrients.

7. The cost of nutrients virtually always falls on the family, while the cost of prescription meds is often covered by public health care or health insurance. We see this discrepancy as

an opportunity to lobby governments to open up plans beyond medications. Shouldn't the pharmaceutical companies lose their monopoly on taxpayer-funded treatments?

8. Given the lower risks associated with minerals and vitamins, a good route to consider might be to try multinutrients *first*. If they don't result in sufficient benefits, consider alternatives.

Anxiety

Anxiety will be covered in much greater detail in chapter 7, especially when we talk about trauma and stress. Overall, there's substantial evidence showing that B vitamins are an effective treatment for stress and anxiety in the general population. A combined vitamin/mineral approach will likely have even larger effects for those who have significant struggles with, or symptoms of, anxiety.

Autism Spectrum Disorder (ASD)

Over sixteen years ago, a small pilot RCT led by Professor James Adams at Arizona State University involving twenty children with ASD was published, showing promising results using a nutrient formula called Spectrum Support™.[5] Those taking the supplement showed improvements in sleep and gastrointestinal problems, with trends suggesting some improved behavior, eye contact, and receptive language. Ten years ago, these researchers followed up with a much larger RCT with 141 children and adults with autism, finding positive effects of a modified version of the formula (then called Syndion™) over a placebo in reducing tantrums and hyperactivity as well as improving receptive language and overall functioning.[6] The formulas evaluated contained twenty-nine nutrients and all participants were monitored for three months.

Then in 2018, these same researchers published an effectiveness trial comparing multinutrients (at this stage called ANRC Essentials Plus™) alongside other nutritional supplements (including EFAs, Epsom salts, carnitine, digestive enzymes) and a gluten-free, dairy-free diet vs. no treatment over a twelve-month period. They observed significantly greater change in the treatment group across many areas of functioning for those who received the comprehensive treatment approach, including improvement in symptoms of ASD, social responsiveness, sensory profile, nonverbal IQ, and aberrant behavior.[7]

A study published by psychiatrist Lewis Mehl-Madrona and his colleagues (including Bonnie) systematically followed forty-four children, some for up to two years, whose families chose to use EMP for the clinical treatment of ASD.[8] Subsequently, these children were matched by age, gender, and symptom severity to forty-four children from the same clinic whose families had chosen conventional meds to treat the symptoms. The multinutrients were superior to medication in reducing both irritability and self-harming behaviors. In fact, self-harm was reduced by 50 percent. Not surprisingly, there were far fewer side effects reported for those on the multinutrients compared with those on meds (33 vs. 214).

Much more research is needed, but as scientists continue to unravel the very real possibility that proper functioning of the gut is somehow involved with ASD, it's a logical assumption that improving nutrition should confer some benefit on these behaviors through increasing the amount of nutrients available for the brain.

Bipolar Disorder

We've both wanted to do randomized controlled trials of people with bipolar disorder, as it can be such a debilitating illness. However, a study Bonnie started in Alberta in the late 1990s eventually had to be abandoned due to the hostile political climate, and Julia has never been able to con-

vince any of the psychiatrists in her city to consider nutrients before medications for bipolar disorder, even within the context of a research study.

All studies on bipolar *symptoms* have been done using one product
only, EMP. There have been numerous open-label trials (studies where
everyone receives the treatment),[9] case studies,[10] and database analyses
in adults[11] and children[12] with bipolar symptoms, all showing much-im-
proved symptoms and a lessened need for the amount of meds required
to maintain symptom control for most of the participants. Some of these
studies reported up to 80 percent of participants showing a substantial reduction in their symptoms. But while the findings have been consistent,
they don't provide data from the RCTs needed to convince mainstream
medicine to consider the power of nutrients in stabilizing this condition.
There is one RCT in progress in the United States, but it's too soon to
provide further information.

How Nutrients Helped Benjy

One of the crossover trials showed on/off control of symptoms in
two boys with severe mood dysregulation.[13] Bonnie has kept in
touch with Benjy, one of the boys, for more than twenty years.

Benjy was twelve years old when his family volunteered
to participate in one of Bonnie's first evaluations of EMP
for mood dysregulation. Benjy was initially diagnosed at
age two with autism, and was re-diagnosed at age four with
pervasive developmental disorder. But the symptoms that
challenged him the most were his irritable temperament and
his explosive outbursts, which became more frequent as he
approached puberty. He began running away from home and
reporting his parents to the police. The drug Adderall brought
some improvement in his attention span, but his emotional
dysregulation did not improve. Before he began taking the

nutrients, his parents chose to discontinue the Adderall; by that time, even a full-time teacher's aide was not enough for Benjy to be able to stay in school, and alternatives were being sought. His teachers reported that he was loud, disruptive, rude, and out of control.

For the duration of the study, his mother (an experienced special education teacher) rated Benjy on a measure of ADHD. Three weeks after beginning the nutrients, there was noticeable improvement in his temper and mood (see graph). When the nutrients were stopped, his mood and temper problems returned to baseline (pre-treatment). Reintroduction of the nutrients resulted in improvements again. (This type of design is sometimes called ABAB, to refer to the on-off-on-off nature of the design.)

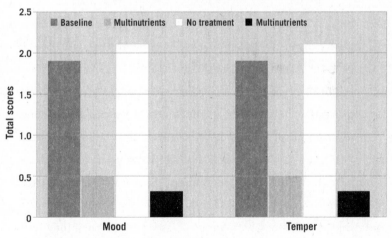

Benjy's Response to Multinutrient Treatment

From *Journal of Child and Adolescent Psychopharmacology* 12, Issue 3, by permission of Mary Ann Liebert, Inc.

What has happened to Benjy since then? Not only was he able to go back to his classes, but he graduated from high school. Now in his early thirties, he lives independently in his own apartment, and remains very close to his entire family. He has become an excellent cook, eats an exceptionally healthy diet, rides his bike everywhere, and gets lots of other exercise, too. In contrast to many people with his history, Benjy looks healthy and very fit.

But here is a critical component to Benjy's success with the multinutrients, which he continues to take: unlike some individuals, especially those with developmental delays and on the autism spectrum, *Benjy knows that he feels and functions better when taking the nutrients.* From a very early age, he made sure he always had a sufficient supply on hand. His insight and adherence with taking the multinutrient formula seem integral to his excellent health.

Depression

One of the challenges of the mood-symptom studies using nutrients in pill form has been that most of them have been done with people who don't have any significant depression when they are recruited to join the studies. Not surprisingly, those studies using people who have little room for improvement have not shown much benefit from additional nutrients.

In addition, most of the studies done on depression have been conducted with only a few nutrients, not a broad spectrum. This distinction is important. At this stage, the findings on many selected nutrients are mixed; some show benefit, but most don't. And one study of two vitamins and two minerals along with omega-3 fatty acids to see if they could prevent the development of depression also highlighted the erroneous thinking in these selective-nutrient studies (not surprisingly, these few nutrients were unable to prevent depression more than placebo).[14]

Clinical trials like these show the problem when studies are done using only a "favorite few" of the nutrients as the treatment. Selecting nutrients in a sort of shotgun manner is not the best way to target complex psychiatric disorders. As described in chapter 2, it makes much more biological sense to use the entire spectrum of minerals and vitamins and other nutrients your brain needs for optimal functioning. These studies also highlight the challenges of adding nutrients on top of medications, a problem discussed in detail in chapter 11.

One study with positive results included 330 adults with major depressive disorder (MDD) who had certain variants of the MTHFR gene.[15] Half got Enlyte (a supplement with folic acid, folinic acid, methylfolate, zinc, magnesium, thiamine, nicotinamide, and B12) and half got a placebo. As you learned in chapter 2, MTHFR variants affect the methylation cycle, so those in the study likely had sluggish methylation cycles already.

Those who got the nutrients had a greater reduction in their depression symptoms compared to those receiving the placebo, with 42 percent remission at eight weeks. This study highlights the possible benefit of gene testing, but we don't know if the same results would have been found in people with normal MTHFR enzyme levels, so we can't generalize these results to all individuals with depression.

Two recent Australian studies have continued to challenge us to think a lot more about the problem of combining a "favorite few" nutrients rather than being guided by biology. Both clinical trials selected a few "key" nutrients that had been found to help with mood disorders when added to medications. Seventy percent were already taking an SSRI (selective serotonin reuptake inhibitor) antidepressant medication but they continued to be symptomatic despite the meds. (Several people had complications during the study because taking serotonin precursors such as 5HTP while using SSRIs could lead to an overproduction of serotonin.)

Both trials had a very large placebo effect and there were no differences between the nutrient and placebo groups. In one, the nutrients studied were five vitamins, two minerals, EPA+DHA (omega-3s), 5HTP, and

SAMe.[16] (5HTP is a precursor in the synthesis of serotonin and thus is believed to boost serotonin levels. SAMe is involved in the methylation cycle, so it might help with sluggish metabolic pathways.) After eight weeks, the groups did not differ. The researchers entitled their paper "More Is Not Merrier," and this study has been cited erroneously as evidence that nutrients in general are ineffective as a treatment for serious mood problems. Similarly, in their second sixteen-week study there was no difference between placebo and a nutrient supplement referred to as a "mitochondrial cocktail," though not all key nutrients important for the citric acid cycle and general brain metabolism were included (there were twelve vitamins but only two minerals — calcium and magnesium).[17] The only conclusion to be drawn from these two studies is that these particular combinations of nutrients in patients of this type were not helpful.

Many of the studies we've told you about are highly controlled with strict inclusion criteria, and they often don't help us know how to apply the information to people in the "real" world. There is one study we want to describe because it tells us about the translation of research into practice. A nonprofit company in Calgary, Alberta, Canada, called Pure North has been offering nutrients along with other holistic advice to Albertans since 2007. They provide a broad range of vitamins, minerals, amino acids, probiotics, and omega-3s at no cost to low-income and homeless people, as well as to anyone who enrolls in their program who pays. They evaluated the effectiveness of their nutrient package for improving mental health by monitoring over 16,000 individuals over a one-year period. Their results were published in 2018, with Julia as a co-author.[18] Half of the respondents showed improvement in their mood at one year. Most notable was that over 90 percent of those who reported severe or extreme depression or anxiety at program entry showed substantial improvement.

Julia's lab is currently running a clinical trial comparing DEN with a placebo for the treatment of symptoms of depression in adults recruited through general medical practices, and it should be finished by 2021.[19]

Hopefully we can continue to shed more light on whether a broad-spectrum approach has a greater effect on symptoms of depression than the selected/favorite-few nutrients approach does.

Pregnancy-Related Mental Health, and Neurodevelopmental Problems in Offspring

Although a number of studies have focused on the prevention of postnatal depression using nutritional supplements, very few have investigated their use for the treatment of anxiety and depression *during* pregnancy. One study showed that a broad-spectrum multivitamin and mineral supplement taken during the preconception period improved symptoms of depression for women with evidence of mood problems.[20] An RCT of Elevit™, a popular multinutrient supplement taken during pregnancy, which contains eleven vitamins and eight minerals, reduced symptoms of depression more than a supplement with just calcium and vitamin D when taken post-delivery in healthy women over a one-month period.[21]

Research that followed the infants of mothers who used multivitamins of any type during pregnancy found that nutrient use was associated with a reduced risk of autism at three years and ADHD at seven years.[22] All other studies have looked at the relationship between *single* nutrients and the risk of neurodevelopmental disorders; for example, low vitamin D can increase the chances of having a child with autism and/or schizophrenia by two- to threefold.[23] The evidence was considered so strong by Dr. Robert Freedman, the editor of the *American Journal of Psychiatry*, that he stated, "As part of comprehensive maternal and fetal care, prenatal nutrient interventions should be further considered as uniquely effective first steps in decreasing risk for future psychiatric and other illnesses in newborn children."[24] If single nutrients are perceived as so important, what impact could a broad spectrum of nutrients have on infant development?

This question led to the NUTRIMUM trial, an ongoing study in Julia's lab that's looking at the role of broad-spectrum multinutrients on a mother's mental health, both during and after pregnancy, and also whether exposure to nutrients during pregnancy has any effect on infant birth and ongoing development.[25] The multinutrient formula is DEN, and the study is expected to be finished by 2021.

Psychosis and Schizophrenia

Dr. Lewis Mehl-Madrona has been a leader in conducting studies of a multinutrient approach to alleviate the suffering of those with psychosis and schizophrenia. These are two of the most severely debilitating and chronic psychiatric problems, with no known cause and no known cure. However, there have been a number of published cases showing the power of broad-spectrum multinutrients in reducing or eliminating psychotic symptoms, and countless other anecdotal stories as well.

Dr. Mehl-Madrona published an interesting analysis of nineteen patients who gradually switched from medications to EMP.[26] The study started off as an RCT with a one-month lead-in: this design provided everyone with EMP in the first month. At the end of the first month, they were supposed to be randomized so half would get the multinutrients and half would get the placebo, but not a single participant was willing to do that because they were already feeling so much better! That finding in itself is extraordinary — all these patients independently balked at losing their multinutrient-related benefits and chose to withdraw from the study rather than risk getting a placebo.

The researchers were forced to change their study design and monitor these participants over two years instead, comparing their progress to thirty-one patients who chose not to participate in any nutrition research. At fifteen months, the group receiving both medication and multinutrients had significantly fewer psychosis symptoms than the medication-only group. This difference was even stronger at the two-year mark. The researchers concluded that a broad-spectrum multinutrient formula was a beneficial long-term adjunct strategy for people with psychotic disorders. When they took the nutrients, they needed smaller doses of their meds to be effective, with fewer side effects.

However, the biggest challenge that we face in giving advice to those who are struggling with psychosis and wanting to try nutrients is that most of them come to us on heavy-duty prescription meds, often under forced treatment.

This is an example of one of the heartbreaking emails we've received over the years: "I am a forty-five-year-old mother of three children. Currently I am under the Mental Health Act, having been diagnosed with schizoaffective disorder and PTSD, and am forced to have the slow-release olanzapine injection every month against my will. If I refuse, my doctor or psychiatric nurse can call the police and have me brought into the hospital. The side effects are dreadful and my quality of life is no good. I have contacted a lawyer and will be appealing against this. Is there anything you could do to help me?"

As you'll see in chapter 11, antipsychotic medications complicate the road to recovery for those who want to take the nutrients, and we strongly encourage anyone who wants to manage their psychosis with nutrition to discuss any changes of medications with their prescriber. There are serious risks associated with stopping medications without supervision, and the clinical advice is to reduce medications very slowly and alongside professional help. Given the number of emails like this that we receive, we really hope psychiatrists will someday take the lead in discovering how to manage successful cross-titrations (meaning gradually introducing nutrients and then gradually reducing medications).

One patient who chose the nutrients to treat psychotic symptoms was a woman named Andri, who wrote about her experience in one of Julia's studies on the Mad in America website (madinamerica.com), the website established by science journalist and author Robert Whitaker following the enormous success of his 2001 book by that name. Andri revealed her extended involvement with psychiatric services, including hospitalizations, medications, and ECT, after she was diagnosed with major depression with psychotic features. Against all medical advice, she chose to try nutrients to manage her symptoms rather than medications. She wrote:

> Once I was on the nutrients, there was an improvement in my "ratings" on the mood questionnaires and interviews I took part in monthly. Less distress ... further spaced-apart "episodes" that I became quicker to recover from, and generally better-regulated emotions. This was hard to trust, initially. My thoughts were still very negative and I would catch myself regularly ruminating on what I had been told: that I just couldn't expect myself to "recover" and stay well without meds, that the stats were against me ... that it wasn't possible.
>
> My newly improved state started to make sense after I reviewed my hospital notes again — this time with a nutrition lens on. They found low potassium, which I learned impacts brain functioning and therefore could contribute to psychosis. I was eventually treated for the low potassium during my admission, but I wonder why they did not start there. I often questioned whether I would have needed invasive "treatments" at all had they first enabled me to gain optimal nutrition, enough rest and time to meaningfully connect with the people around me. So I kept at it, continued the trial — which was open label by that stage — and continued my yoga routine, gratitude journaling, meaningful work, spending time with my family, preparing for the birth, and working out a plan to manage on a practical level, which resulted in the decision to enlist the help of an au pair. The brain fog started to clear, and without it, problem solving and decision making became a lot easier.

By the time my baby was born earlier this year, I was elated. I was a third-time beginner . . . yet I was wiser. I had another chance to grow in my competence and capacity to maintain a well state through another significant life change.

Since coming off meds and learning to live well, I have few regrets . . .

One important part of this story is that Andri's journey to wellness was not just about the nutrients, but a holistic change in her life, including a good diet, meditation, yoga, and social connections.

The Story of Ginger

Bonnie: In 1997 I was asked to find a psychiatrist at the University of Calgary to evaluate a woman with a history of schizophrenia.

Ginger was a woman living on a farm in southern Alberta. She was diagnosed with schizophrenia in 1984 and was taking several medications. She was unable to function but lived on the farm with her husband, who took care of her. For at least five years, Ginger had spent her days mostly in bed, terrified by the bugs she felt crawling on her skin and saw climbing up the walls. There were many days when she did not get up except to eat or go to the bathroom.

Ginger's husband had heard about the development of a nutrient treatment of mental symptoms by Tony Stephan and David Hardy, the founders of the Alberta companies, something they were then calling the "Quad Program" (it consisted of pills and liquid minerals from four different bottles). This was before they had formed Truehope Nutritional Support and developed their own product.

Ginger's husband decided to give some of the nutrients to his wife, beginning in late December 1996. Ginger improved a great deal over two months, and the family was able to significantly reduce her meds. By four months she was symptom-free and was once again participating in household activities. She was so well that they decided to take a road trip to a neighboring province to visit family. While they were there, they ran out of nutrients and Ginger began to decline. Tony and David had the idea that they would provide more nutrients to Ginger at no cost if she would agree to be seen by a Calgary psychiatrist to assess her pre- and post-treatment with the goal of publishing a case report. So they called and asked me to find a psychiatrist to do that.

I wasn't sure if I could find someone. But I phoned a newly trained psychiatrist who I thought would be open; I will call her Dr. M. She agreed to assess Ginger, who was brought to Calgary for the evaluation after being off the nutrients for four months. Dr. M called me afterward and said that Ginger suffered from severe chronic schizophrenia so she did not see why we were trying to help her (in other words, her case was hopeless).

Nevertheless, Ginger was restarted on the nutrients (still the "Quad Program") at month number eleven in the graph, and again she responded well. Dr. M was amazed, of course, at her next evaluation of Ginger. So then I offered to help Dr. M write it up as a case report for publication, and I'll never forget her response: "Bonnie, this would really hurt my reputation. I can't be seen as having an interest in minerals and vitamins."

The lack of interest from so many mental health practitioners we have encountered over the years—and in some cases like Ginger's, a clear lack of intellectual curiosity—has been a major stumbling block, both in carrying out further research

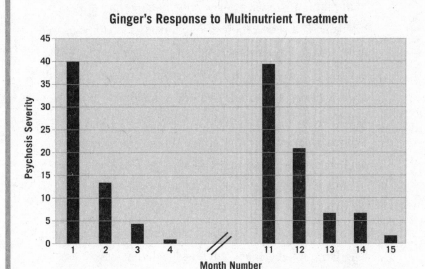

Ginger's Response to Multinutrient Treatment

and in supporting people to transition from meds to nutrients. The case studies we have observed are so rich in opportunity to reverse a chronic and devastating illness. We owe it to these people to carry out the type of research that can offer a real alternative to what their current options provide.

The Takeaway

1. The scientific evidence is strong, such that all health professionals should consider diet and nutrients as a frontline treatment for psychiatric disorders. Nutrition is not magic, but it should be one of the first tools clinicians reach for from their toolbox.
2. Many studies have shown that supplementing with a single nutrient at a time or a "favorite few" often given alongside medications is not as effective as a broad-spectrum

multinutrient approach. As you learned in chapter 2, our brains need a wide variety of minerals and vitamins as well as essential fatty acids. Frankly, if you are trying to resolve— not just improve—a mental disorder, the research shows it's a waste of research funds to study one nutrient or a select few at a time.

3. The most powerful proven effect of the broad-spectrum approach is improved ability to regulate emotions, which can then lead to improvements in other problematic areas, like mood, anxiety, irritability, and aggression.

4. For those with ADHD who benefit and stay on the nutrients long term, improvement can be expected across all areas of functioning including mood, anxiety, and ADHD symptoms.

5. Multinutrient supplements might also have a profound effect on people with autism spectrum disorder. Also promising are the published data that relate to psychotic disorders. The promising results thus far should encourage scientists to continue to investigate this treatment.

6. Many people who suffer from different mental health conditions can lower the dosage of their prescription meds when they take broad-spectrum multinutrients. This suggests that a healthier brain needs less medication, which leads to fewer of the often debilitating side effects that make people unhappy with their treatment.

7. Much more research needs to be done—and funding provided for comprehensive studies and clinical trials—but the results are encouraging. We seem to be on the verge of providing an entirely new answer to an age-old question: What causes mental illness?

6

TACKLING LIFE'S CHALLENGES WITH SUPPLEMENTS

LIFE IS FULL OF significant challenges for all of us. Many of these challenges don't necessarily fall into a psychiatric diagnostic category, but can lead to problems at work, problems with your friends and loved ones, and reduced overall quality of life.

In this chapter, we'll cover these issues. Want to quit smoking? Struggling with sleep? Looking for a natural solution to PMS? Wondering whether there are nutrients to help slow cognitive decline? There is some research we can share that might help resolve some of these life challenges.

Reducing Addiction

Smoking and other addictions present a huge public health problem. They're often treated with psychiatric medications, either antidepressants or pain meds. So while smokers might be confused about seeing their lifestyle choice in this chapter, about 14 percent of Americans are smokers — and every one of them knows how hard it is to quit.

Julia: I first met Brian when he was twenty years old. He had been in and out of psychiatric services and had received a number of diagnostic labels, including ADHD, MDD, and panic disorder. He had a menial job in an advertising agency and he was often off "sick" and unable to manage a full working day. He used both marijuana and cigarettes daily; he said they helped him cope and simply "get through the day." As with so many people I see, he had been tried on a multitude of medications, including stimulants, antidepressants, and antipsychotics. However, he had stopped them all as they "just didn't help" and he hated the side effects like drowsiness and feeling numb and irritable.

Brian participated in one of our earliest studies, an ABAB trial for youth with mood dysregulation. That meant he was on the multinutrient formula (EMP) for eight weeks, stopped it for eight weeks, and then went back on it while we followed him for an additional four months.

We noted substantial changes in Brian's mood within a week. He went from being in the severe range on a measure of depression to being in remission. After two weeks on the pills, Brian told us that he could sit through an entire movie, which he had never been able to do previously, and he reported being able to "focus on one thing at a time." By six weeks on the nutrients, Brian's partner reported that he was more motivated, less "on the go," getting to work on time, less paranoid, less wound up, and more "laid back."

At eight weeks, Brian stopped by my office to tell me how great he felt. It was in this conversation that I learned that Brian had quit smoking cigarettes the previous week (he told me he just didn't crave them anymore) and was no longer using marijuana on a daily basis. When Brian first told me he had decided to quit smoking, I was actually dismayed. That's because when conducting research, you only want to manipulate one variable at a time and I was concerned that his symptoms would return as he withdrew from cigarettes and marijuana! But these lifestyle changes are all part of research, just like when people go on vacation, experience major traumas, or get divorced in the middle of a clinical trial. It all goes with the territory.

Brian was then instructed to stop the nutrients (as per the study's protocol) and within a week, he was feeling more stressed out and had resumed smoking and using more marijuana. He had also been late to work due to sleeping through his alarm, and was having difficulties in focusing at both work and home; getting distracted and quickly losing interest in things; being fidgety, disorganized, and forgetful; and starting tasks but not finishing them.

During this off-phase, symptoms of depression also returned, placing Brian in the moderate-severe clinical range. He was experiencing more mood swings in that he would get agitated every couple of days and annoyed at his partner and friends over small things. His sleep had also worsened; he felt tired during the day and had to "drag himself out of bed." His partner stated that Brian was "more snappy, wound up, and does not leave the house."

Brian then went back on the nutrients. Within three weeks, his mood and sleep were back to normal. He described himself as not on edge anymore and having no difficulties with concentration. At this point in time, there was a 7.1 earthquake in Christchurch and Brian's reaction was monitored. He coped really well with it, helped out with the recovery effort, and didn't experience any deterioration in his anxiety or mood. At four months, he was in remission, and not smoking anything. Brian's experience inspired my lab to run a much larger controlled clinical trial investigating whether nutrients can help people quit cigarettes. One of my former Master's students, Rachel Tauamiti (née Harrison), also published Brian's case as part of her thesis.[1]

The idea that there might be a link between smoking and nutrition is not even a blip on the radar for most researchers or clinicians. We know that smokers typically have poorer diets than nonsmokers, but until Julia's lab ran a study, no one had investigated whether ensuring optimal nutrition levels when attempting to quit smoking might be relevant and even helpful in the quitting process. Back in 1956, biochemist Roger Williams reported a 50 percent success rate in reversing a different substance abuse (alcohol) by improving nutrient intake, and he speculated that much of the dependence on such substances was due to nutrient insufficiency: "It appears that the uncontrolled craving for alcohol in certain individuals is a nutritional deficiency disease. I have had intimate contact with several individuals (and less intimate contact with many more) who initially had this craving to an extreme degree, but who, by eating more wisely and taking nutritional supplements, have had their craving completely abolished so that now they behave as individuals who never were alcoholics; they drink little or none as they wish."

A few preliminary studies in the 1980s also showed the potential of multinutrients in helping people overcome various forms of addiction, including alcohol and cocaine. Since 1990, no other researchers had delved into the role nutrients could play in overcoming addiction.

One of Julia's former PhD students, Dr. Pip Reihana, decided to explore this idea in greater depth with a controlled study. Given that tobacco smoking is often used to cope with stress and multinutrients have been well established to reduce stress, Pip wondered whether taking multinutrients would moderate the stress of withdrawal and increase the chance of a successful quit attempt.

This study is the first known RCT investigating the impact of a broad-spectrum multinutrient formula (DEN) to reduce or stop cigarettes altogether.[2] She recruited 107 smokers and randomized them to take either the multinutrients or a placebo, and all participants received assistance from Quit New Zealand, also known as Quitline, which offers online support and ideas on how to distract, delay, and decrease cigarette consumption.

Based on all of those participants who received the full intervention (pills + Quitline), regardless of whether they completed the study, we found that 42 percent of the multinutrient group achieved full abstinence for twelve weeks versus 23 percent of the placebo group. In fact, the multinutrients were comparable or better to other smoking cessation treatments, but with far fewer side effects. This quit rate is higher than that observed with the drug Champix (twelve-week quit rate: 22 percent) as well as Nicotine Replacement Therapy + Quitline (twelve-week quit rate: 26 percent), the treatments for smoking cessation that the New Zealand government currently pays for. Even more amazing was that our placebo was about as good as these medication options funded by the government!

Also notable was the finding that those who received the multinutrient formula smoked fewer cigarettes during the quit-attempt phase and up to four weeks post-quitting.

Still, we need to be cautious about over-interpreting these results. We had a high dropout rate (58 percent) and the sample size was small relative to drug company–funded studies. Staying off nicotine is difficult, and it was not surprising that many relapsed over the course of the three-month study.

This novel study tentatively supports the use of nutrients to assist with quitting smoking and to reduce the consumption of cigarettes, particularly during the acute stage of withdrawal. We hope these promising results lead to further funding and investment in larger studies. Who wouldn't want to use a nutrient approach to help quit smoking, given all the other health benefits of this treatment?

Aggression and Explosive Rage

The benefit of using nutrients to reduce antisocial behaviors and aggression has been known for decades! It's astonishing that this knowledge isn't routinely implemented in prisons, where violence is a huge problem. As it is in many psychiatric inpatient units in hospitals around the world.

Wouldn't everyone want prisoners, patients, and children to be less aggressive?

We have both published studies showing the reduction in aggression in children given a broad spectrum of multinutrients.[3] We have also both seen countless kids who were so emotionally dysregulated that they would flare up without warning, becoming physically violent, throwing things, breaking toys, and biting and hitting other children. These are the kids who can be fine one minute and then completely out of control the next, with temper tantrums lasting for hours. The parents always report that nothing seems to work, and they are often told to take a parenting class. We *love* seeing those kids because the nutrients can have such a profound effect on these behaviors, and often quite quickly.

This is what happened to a lovely little boy named Liam.

Bonnie: I went to answer the front door and was not surprised to see Peter there with an envelope in his hand. Peter was providing some financial information to my husband and me, and he had offered to drop off some papers. I invited him in for coffee even though we barely knew each other, but I sensed that Peter was very, very tired. I did not need to probe — just a simple "Is work very overwhelming right now?" type of question opened the floodgates. Peter was indeed stressed and tired, but not because of work. His home life was unraveling and he did not know what to do about it.

Peter and his wife had two children, a six-year-old boy and a four-year-old girl. The boy, Liam, was having meltdown after meltdown at home. Oddly, the school reported that he was a lovely, sweet child with no emotional challenges. Peter and his wife accepted that they must not be parenting as well as they should, and they took courses in child management and participated in family therapy. Nothing was working. On a typical day Liam had two or three major rage attacks at home.

I asked about Liam's diet, after explaining a bit about my research. I was somewhat surprised to learn that he was the opposite of a picky eater: he would eat anything his parents prepared, and they tried to serve healthy food. Nevertheless, it seemed that it would be worth a try to give Liam one of the broad-spectrum formulas.

Unfortunately, Liam had not yet learned to swallow pills. I gave Peter the link to my pill-swallowing training video (research4kids.ucalgary.ca/pillswallowing), but really wanted to get him started on something quickly with the hopes of reducing the stress in this family. I suggested they go to a health food store and buy a liquid mineral formula. I had no particular brand to recommend (to the best of my knowledge, none of them has yet been studied by independent scientists), so I suggested they buy whichever one came in the smallest bottle. That way, if there was no benefit, they would not have wasted much money.

Peter told me that since he was very data-oriented, he was going to start a spreadsheet to keep track of Liam's meltdowns. I thought that was a good idea, but I reminded him that they were not part of any research study, there was no consent form, and that I was just offering some advice as a friend.

Peter created his spreadsheet and started his son on the liquid minerals. The result: Liam has not had another long meltdown since then —for over three years! The change was not instantly perfect: Liam still occasionally began to work up to a tantrum for several days, but in each case he was able to calm himself down and self-regulate his emotions.

I am not comfortable suggesting that a child take only minerals without vitamins, because of how they work together in our brains, as you know from chapter 2. So I also encouraged the family to use the training video and get Liam to be able to swallow pills. He pretty quickly became a champion pill swallower, and they switched him to one of the Alberta broad-spectrum formulas. Now, three years later, Peter says that if they forget to provide the minerals on too many occasions, or if Liam is especially overtired, he still has fifteen-minute meltdowns, but they are mild and brief compared to the hour-long loss of emotional control in the pre-supplement days.

Even Bees Become Less Aggressive from Minerals!

There are lots of reasons to look at other creatures on our planet for clues about the importance of dietary nutrients. In Alberta, the need for additional minerals for farm animals behaving aggressively is well established, and is what led David Hardy to think of adding nutrients to treat the mental health problems in Tony Stephan's children, as we described in the Introduction.[4] In the laboratory, scientists have repeatedly shown that low intake of some minerals results in aggressive behavior in rodent models.

So it should come as no surprise to find out that even insects such as honeybees are affected by minerals. In a 2020 issue of a magazine entitled *Eco Farming Daily,* a professional beekeeper in Utah described how he eliminated colony collapse disorder (CCD) and reduced aggression in his hives. As he pointed out, bees are now exposed to large amounts of herbicides and pesticides, which destroy the healthy microbes in their digestive systems and weaken their immune systems. In addition, the vast majority of food producers do not restore their fields with the full range of trace elements that have been depleted, which then decreases the mineral consumption by bees. Over the course of four years, this beekeeper eliminated CCD by spraying his hives with a probiotic and an array of minerals. One of the most remarkable observations he made was that the difference in his hives was audible: when they were sprayed with the probiotic and mineral supplement, the bees were much quieter. "They are calmer and much easier to work with. They are less excitable when we move them around or need to get into the hive. In fact, we don't use smoke

> anymore when we work with our bees. Instead, we just spray
> some [of the supplement] onto the open hive and the bees
> settle right down."

Internationally, there have been case studies, open-label studies, and multiple RCTs showing that multinutrients can successfully reduce aggression and violent incidents across a range of populations from delinquent children to incarcerated adults. The earliest controlled trial was over twenty years ago, when California researchers found that giving children a broad array of minerals such as calcium, magnesium, and zinc along with vitamins such as thiamine, riboflavin, and folate in doses at least equivalent to, and sometimes higher than, the RDA (recommended dietary allowance) resulted in a 28 percent greater decrease in rule violations at school compared with those receiving the placebo.[5]

Another RCT conducted by these same researchers showed that giving antisocial schoolchildren aged six to twelve a broad spectrum of nutrients yielded even better results.[6] The forty children in the experimental group who were given a multinutrient supplement exhibited 47 percent fewer antisocial behaviors requiring discipline than the forty children who received a placebo. The types of behaviors the researchers monitored included threats, fighting, vandalism, defiance, endangering others, and disorderly conduct. Some European studies continued to demonstrate the benefits of additional nutrients for aggression, with similar effects on violent behaviors within prisons.[7]

The implications of these studies are profound. A simple intervention using broad-spectrum multinutrient supplements could have *wide-reaching* effects on our schools and on young offenders.

All the studies show that multinutrient treatment may decrease aggressive behavior, providing enough evidence for policy changes within prisons. It is disheartening that this research has been around for over two decades — yet it hasn't influenced how we address aggressive and violent behavior in children and adults.

Rather than try to solve the problem by improving the nutrient intake of these most vulnerable people, government-run boards of health tend to react by using heavy-duty meds for sedation as well as hiring more guards. We would better understand their reluctance to use nutrients if there was no evidence about them . . . but there is!

Until this changes, we will continue to get messages like this one, a recent email to Julia:

Hi Julia,

In brief, my daughter is six years old, and I have been struggling with her since she was about two and a half years old. She has poor emotional regulation, physical and verbal outbursts, fails to follow any direction from authority figures — the list goes on — and more recently, since starting school, she is struggling to concentrate and focus on learning.

Teachers have had difficulty with her concentration, defiance, and "argy bargys" with other children, which they have mentioned to me. They have said not to give up getting her help, because it is now affecting her learning, and something is definitely not right.

I have taken her to naturopaths, spent hundreds in health shops, and attended parenting courses as advised by the Ministry of Education. We sold our home and I changed jobs, decreasing my work hours, as I was told it was attention-seeking behavior and it was all my fault she was the way she was for being too busy. I knew it wasn't, but I was desperate and open to trying anything and everything.

A referral was made to the child mental health service but it was declined, as they have no staff and are too busy. After all of this we had no improvement. I was concerned for my daughter to the point that I have now been paying for private psychology sessions.

I strongly believe my daughter has ODD [oppositional defiant disorder] with some ADHD traits. I am just at a loss for how to help her now, but it seems people have found your micronutrients helpful.

I am open to giving anything a go. I have two other children who are being exposed to this awful behavior and it truly breaks my heart. My two-and-a-half-year-old son is now learning some of these behaviors, which I wanted to avoid.

Any advice will be greatly appreciated. I would even be willing to fly down and meet with you if this is better suited.

At this stage all we can do when we receive these messages is send them the information we've gathered about this treatment approach and how to access it, and then hope that this will help them on their journey.

Cognitive Impairment

We want to briefly touch on this fairly large body of research as it overlaps with psychological functioning — good mental acuity can have a positive effect on mood and vice versa. The small but positive impact of additional nutrients on the academic performance of schoolchildren has been known for several decades.[8] Interestingly, a review of this literature came to a conclusion similar to ours with respect to mental health — studies using supplementation with a single or restricted range of vitamins have mixed results, while evidence from studies using a broader range of nutrients shows stronger effects on cognitive and psychological functioning.[9]

More recently, some researchers have started delving into whether additional nutrients can help slow cognitive decline. Given our aging population, this is an extremely important area for study. This is another situation where the focus has been on B vitamins because of their known importance for the methylation cycle you learned about in chapter 2. If the cycle doesn't run smoothly, one result is an increase in homocysteine, an amino acid that, when consistently elevated, has been found to be associated with oxidative stress, a risk factor for cognitive decline, dementia, and Alzheimer's disease in older persons.[10] Increasing vitamin B intake has been shown to reduce homocysteine levels, which is why treatment studies have tended to be on B vitamins.

A natural part of aging is neuron loss, which is called brain atrophy. Of course we all want to minimize our brain atrophy as much as possible! One randomized trial (called VITACOG) done at the University of Oxford found some remarkable effects on brain atrophy in people who took a relatively high dose of daily B vitamins.[11] The participants were 150 seniors over the age of seventy with mild cognitive impairment, who were given either B vitamins (0.8 mg folic acid, 20 mg of vitamin B6, and 0.5 mg of vitamin B12) or a placebo for two years. The results showed that those who had high homocysteine levels when they started the study, and were lucky enough to be given the B vitamins, experienced slowed whole-brain atrophy by 53 percent, slowed atrophy of specific brain regions by 90 percent, and slowed, or stopped, further cognitive decline. If research like this can be replicated, the use of nutrients like B vitamins to decrease our risk for dementia would be a promising and affordable option.[12]

Hopefully, all the research being done on cognitive issues will also help those who struggle with the effects of a traumatic brain injury. A young man in Christchurch, Sam Johnson, who is a bit of a national hero in New Zealand as he is the founder of the Student Volunteer Army, suffered a TBI after he was accidentally hit in the head by a hedge trimmer. In a public posting on Facebook, he said: ". . . at University recently, I see Professor Julia Rucklidge who does research on how high doses of micronutrients can support brain function for head injury recovery. I am testing it out and so far, I'm amazed. My ability to function has increased dramatically with headaches reduced, less irritability, stronger ability to focus, and longer length of time on a screen . . . Thank you Julia for your life's work exploring this hugely important area."

Bonnie published a case study of a man who used nutrients to assist with the residual emotional effects of a TBI.[13] Tristan was a twenty-seven-year-old munitions specialist working for the British military, doing dangerous tasks such as defusing bombs. One day in 2005 he was walking down the street and a drunk driver drove onto the sidewalk, hitting him and throwing him against a brick wall. He sustained injuries to his brain, as well as numerous fractures to his body. He was in intensive care requiring ventilation for two and a half weeks, transferred to a rehabilitation center for eighteen months, and then followed for six years by a community support worker/counselor.

Though Tristan's physical injuries eventually healed well, he was left with extremely dysregulated emotions, where he would sometimes lose control of his temper in a flash. A psychiatric report five and a half years post-trauma stated that Tristan's continued mood changes and aggressive outbursts would continue to be barriers to complete rehabilitation. The psychiatrist felt that "the continued nature of the symptoms so many years after his accident suggested that there was little prospect of further change . . ." and that Tristan's situation was expected to be "permanent."

Tristan had been medication-free for several years while searching for a natural treatment, as he wanted to avoid psychiatric medications. He read about broad-spectrum multinutrients to treat mood dysregulation, irritability, and explosive rage, and he asked to start a trial with them while monitoring his response. By then, he was thirty-five, eight years post-injury, and still afraid to go into a grocery store because if someone accidentally bumped into him, he might "deck him" before being able to control his violent reaction.

A measure of mood instability from a common rating scale was used to

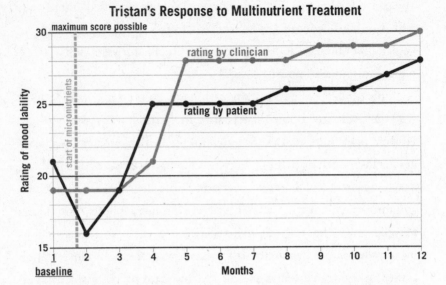

From *Annals of Psychiatry and Mental Health* 4, Issue 5, under Open Access (CC BY 4.0) from JSci-Med Central

evaluate Tristan's mood stability for a few weeks before treatment (called baseline) and then for twelve months after beginning EMP. Tristan and his counselor, who had known him for six years, both scored him monthly, but they hid their ratings from each other to avoid biasing each other. Someone else took the ratings and graphed them as shown. As you can see, at the end of twelve months Tristan approached the maximum score of 30, indicating excellent control of his mood.

It is interesting that the time it took for Tristan to improve was very similar to what we often see in people with irritability and aggression not associated with TBI. Tristan himself reported that he actually felt "something" change within two weeks of starting EMP, but he was not sufficiently confident that it was "real" until the four-month evaluation, when he assigned himself a much higher score.

We think the takeaway from Tristan's experience is, as we say several times in this book, that the diagnostic category is not what is important, because no matter what the diagnosis, the broad-spectrum multinutrients help with emotion regulation — controlling irritability, anger, and mood. Interestingly, basic laboratory research on EMP has also found a significant impact when it was given to lab animals with early-life brain lesions.[14] Nutrient supplementation resulted in recovery of learning and motor skills, and a significant regrowth of the previously removed brain tissue. This animal research is certainly compelling and, along with these case studies, suggests an interesting avenue for assisting recovery from TBI.

Premenstrual Syndrome (PMS)

Before you wonder why this category is here, you should know that PMS regularly affects 20 to 30 percent of all women, and 1.2 to 6.4 percent will experience an even more severely symptomatic form known as premenstrual dysphoric disorder. PMDD includes symptoms of severe depression, mood swings, anxiety, and other symptoms — which is why we've included it in this chapter. Given the average woman will have about five hundred periods over her lifetime, that is a lot of suffering! The most likely treatment a woman will receive for these debilitating symptoms will be an oral contraceptive pill, other hormonal treatment, or antidepressants.

From the beginning of our research on broad-spectrum multinutrients, many women told us that their PMS improved while taking the supplement for another condition. We were intrigued to find that there is a product called Optivite™, the first multivitamin/multimineral supplement formulated to treat PMS — and it's been available for PMS sufferers since the mid-1980s! Who knew? The studies on Optivite™ have all been funded by the company that makes the product, and hence we need to be mindful of that potential conflict of interest, but the reported 50 percent reduction of PMS complaints in the first one to three months taking the formula was encouraging.[15]

Previous research had also been published on vitamin B6 alone for PMS.[16] So one of Julia's former PhD students, Dr. Hāna Retallick-Brown, led an RCT comparing vitamin B6 to EMP in eighty women with PMS. This means the study was comparing two treatments to determine if one was better than the other.

Her study showed that both treatments were extremely effective for PMS; 72 percent of the EMP and 60 percent of the vitamin B6 group were in *remission* for PMS symptoms after three cycles.[17] This is a truly remarkable finding, because it is such a cheap and easy intervention with no side effects. No prescription antidepressant can make that claim.

In addition, the women who took EMP during this study showed a greater improvement than the B6 group in health-related quality of life. Women with PMS often have a very hard time feeling good about anything when the symptoms hit — they're often less productive, less efficient, moodier, and don't want to participate in their usual activities at work and with friends and loved ones. Anyone who's ever suffered from debilitating PMS can certainly relate!

Unfortunately, the subgroup of women with PMDD was not large enough to confirm the superiority of EMP treatment, but there was a clear clinical advantage for those who took the broad-spectrum supplement over vitamin B6 alone. They had a much larger reduction in their PMS symptoms. Given there are very few effective treatments for PMDD, this finding is worthy of further research.

Sleep

Sleep is vital to human functioning and well-being; nevertheless, insomnia, the persistent inability to get sleep of sufficient length and quality, is a common problem among adults and one of the most prevalent contemporary health problems, estimated to affect 12 to 15 percent of the adult population and as many as 50 percent of clients in primary healthcare settings. Insomnia is often seen in conjunction with other health issues, like obesity and cardiovascular disease, and many mental health symptoms, such as anxiety and depression. People with insomnia are likely to take more medications, consume more healthcare resources, miss work more often, and have more work-related and motor vehicle accidents.

There are treatments available — meds tend to be the first go-to treatment — but the problem is that the meds can be addictive and people develop tolerance very quickly, so they need to increase their dose in order to get the same effect. The addiction to the insomnia drug can become worse than the problem it was trying to fix!

As we've already mentioned, we've found in our studies that when we target the treatment to one problem (like ADHD), we often hear about benefits in other areas (like sleep). So, Julia's lab decided to put it to the test and design a study to see if a broad-spectrum multinutrient formula could improve sleep. And it did.

Joanna Lothian, as part of her Master's thesis, followed seventeen people over eight weeks using a multinutrient treatment (Optimal Balance®, a variation of DEN).[18] Participants took the nutrients at breakfast and lunchtime to avoid the energizing effect of the nutrients at night. She used a controlled lead-in time (different people started the nutrients at different times) as a clever way to reduce the placebo effect. Although the sample was small, the benefits were large and robust. All of the following improved: time to drop off to sleep, the number of night awakenings, and sleep quality. And along with improved sleep, there were also observations of improved coping with stress, less anxiety, and better mood.

If nutrients are found to be helpful for sleep, they will usually be a better choice than meds, which are associated with dependence and side effects. Chronic insomnia as well as the other life challenges we touched on in this chapter can lead to debilitating stress. As you'll see in the next chapter, nutrients can have an amazing ability to mitigate the effects of some of life's challenges.

The Takeaway

1. The studies have been small, but there is hope that multinutrient supplements might help smokers cut back or be able to quit for good. Because people report that the nutrients reduce cravings, research for other addictive substances should be carried out.
2. Since the benefits of using broad-spectrum multinutrients to reduce antisocial behaviors and aggression have been known for many years, they should be readily available for use for children with behavior problems, in psychiatric hospitals, and in prisons. *Should* being the operative word!
3. Some studies have been reported on cognitive decline and traumatic brain injuries with promising results. It's hoped that nutrient supplements will be studied further to see if they can help stave off dementia, and broad-spectrum multinutrients will be investigated in future research for people who have experienced TBIs.
4. Nutrients have been shown to help alleviate debilitating PMS symptoms in up to two-thirds of women. Instead of taking antidepressants, trying nutrient supplements first might be very helpful to mitigate symptoms and avoid the need for medication, although more research is needed to prove this for certain.
5. We have documented improvement of sleep with broad-spectrum multinutrient treatment in one study. More research is needed, but it is worth considering if you are one of the millions of insomniacs!

7

IMPROVING RESILIENCE TO TRAUMA AND STRESS WITH SUPPLEMENTS

NATURAL DISASTERS HAVE TAKEN place on earth for as long as this planet has been in existence, but when they arrive unexpectedly, the traumatic impact can be especially severe. Hurricanes and tornadoes usually come with some form of warning so that both physical and psychological preparations can be made. Earthquakes, fires, pandemics, explosions, and the wholly unnatural disaster of terrorist shootings, on the other hand, almost always arrive with a shocking, terrifying jolt. This makes treatment of the aftermath — and the post-traumatic stress that comes with it — even more difficult. And with the increasing number of extreme weather events occurring as a consequence of climate change, we need to ensure that our brains are prepared to manage the stress that will come along with it.

The brain deals with trauma in a specific way, so in this chapter we are going to describe how the very worst of sudden, life-changing circumstances need not result in lingering emotional devastation. Our most current research shows the powerful effect of nutrient supplementation when used by survivors of a traumatic event — because nutrients are so vital to improve resilience to stress, trauma, and natural disasters.

We have both worked with many victims and survivors of tragedies who were amazed at how much better they felt by taking a daily supplement for only a few weeks, especially when other more conventional forms of post-trauma support had failed. It is discouraging that a simple, cost-effective solution to the long-term effects of trauma is still unknown to the public — everyone who needs and deserves all possible resources to help them cope. It also shows how a solution that works so well for people under extreme stress can work for you, even if your stress is not due to a sudden catastrophe but to ongoing challenges in your life.

The Brain's Response to Trauma

When a traumatic event occurs, our immediate response is dictated by the all-too-familiar fight/flight response: the clenching in your gut, the goosebumps across your body, the sudden leap of your heart. Some of us might feel flushed, others cold. Some start to shake, and others find themselves stiff and frozen. Usually the mind starts to race, but sometimes it goes blank.

All of these are features of the stress response, one of the most fundamental in the human body. The stress response is also not uniquely human. We can easily identify a threatened dog, a scared cat, a squirrel frozen in the center of the road. This fight/flight reaction aims to keep us safe from harm, vigilant to potential threat, and able to protect others. It's an evolutionarily primitive system designed to ensure our survival when faced with something that is either real or perceived to be life-threatening.

The fight/flight response system releases the stress hormones adrenaline and cortisol, resulting in a cascade of physiological changes that prepare us to either fight the threat or run away. Changes that occur include the digestive system getting turned off, blood being redirected to muscles, and muscle tension increasing to prepare for extra speed and strength in case you have to flee. When cortisol is released, it creates a boost in energy through increased release of sugar. These physiological changes are essential to get us to safety.

What happens when the threat is gone? Or is still ongoing, as people around the world experienced during the COVID-19 pandemic? The psychological distress people feel during prolonged trauma and following a traumatic event is unpredictable. It can vary from anxiety and fear-based symptoms to depression, dissociation, and extreme irritability. Some people also experience intrusive thoughts or flashbacks associated with the trauma that can be incredibly disturbing and distressing. They might avoid anything that could trigger memories of the event as well as end up in a permanently hypervigilant state as they constantly scan their environment for possible signs of further danger. Others seem to get through completely unscathed.

These symptoms make a lot of sense as they are all designed to prevent a reoccurrence of the life-threatening event. The problem is that over time, the symptoms can end up severely compromising day-to-day functioning and having a huge effect on your quality of life. When these symptoms become problematic over time, we refer to them as post-traumatic stress disorder (PTSD).

Rates of PTSD can vary depending on the trauma, but surveys indicate that about 7 percent of the population as a whole have experienced PTSD at some point in their life, with about 3.5 percent experiencing it over the last year.[1] PTSD incidence following a disaster can range from 30 to 60 percent of those exposed and can persist for two years post-event for up to one-third of those affected.[2] Some people continue to experience the symptoms for years, even decades. This means that PTSD currently affects millions and millions of people. It is an enormous public health issue.

It's hard to predict who will be vulnerable to ongoing problems associated with chronic arousal and who will be resilient. There are, however, a few known factors that increase the chances of having a prolonged stress response, including severity of injury to self and important others, social support, age, personality factors, emotional states, level of destruction of one's home and place of business, and general loss of resources. Genetics and early life experiences might also play a role, causing excessive levels of anxiety in situations that objectively don't call for such a response. Perhaps one of your parents was anxious, and, from an early age, you observed this significant person modeling anxious responses to possibly non-threatening situations. This can inadvertently teach us to respond in the same way. Or perhaps you have been through traumatic and dangerous situations that have sensitized your body and brain to be hypervigilant to danger at all times, on the constant lookout to keep you safe. Some scientists also point to modern society, with our high stress levels, financial difficulties, social media overuse, and reduced social support heightening our anxiety response to a state beyond what is reasonable or optimal.

One factor that has been overlooked in all of this research is the *adequacy of the food and nutrient environment* to meet the needs of a brain under threat.

In chapter 2, we explained the Triage Theory and discussed how nature ensures that micronutrient-dependent functions required for short-term survival (like the fight/flight response) are protected at the expense of longer-term functions (like concentration or regulation of emotions). In other words, in a crisis, most nutrients that we consume in our food will be redirected to the fight/flight response, leaving very little for the rest of our body to operate. You can imagine that if the fight/flight response is being constantly triggered — either because of repeated threats (like earthquake aftershocks) or reminders — then your nutrients are going to get depleted. If we don't replenish them, then it makes perfect sense that our psychological symptoms will become more and more difficult to manage.

One other important thing that we do know is that people tend to eat more poorly in the wake of a disaster. Quite often, access to fresh foods following a natural disaster is more difficult. And then on top of that, the stress response imposes high nutritional needs — which potentially take precedence over other biological needs — further compounding the problem. Not to mention that many people turn to comfort (and not particularly nutritious) foods when they are very stressed.

You can see how outside stress begets even more internal stress for your brain and body! Just when you need even more nutrients to help you cope, it becomes harder to get them. This is a double whammy during the post-disaster period, when physical and psychological resilience is crucial to help you recover.

Dealing with the Trauma of a Pandemic

For years, epidemiologists and virologists have been warning about the lethal effects of a global pandemic, yet no one was able to precisely predict the monster that became COVID-19. Millions of people have been infected by this virus and countless thousands have died; as with the Spanish flu pandemic of 1918–19, the exact mortality rate will never be known, since so many countries have undercounted the victims. The global economy, education, entertainment, travel—even plans for the future—have all been disrupted.

As this pandemic is unfolding in real time during the writing of this book, we can see the effect it is having on the mental health of adults, teenagers, and children who have had every aspect of their lives upended. According to a US Census Bureau Household Pulse Survey from May–June 2020, the pre-pandemic 25 percent rate of depression in the United States had doubled to 50 percent. A recent article highlighted the possible escalation of the mental health crisis looming ahead as a consequence of COVID-19, including substantial increases in anxiety and depression, loneliness, substance use, and domestic violence.[3] Escalating uncertainty about the virus further compounds stress.

And as UN Secretary-General António Guterres said to *Time* magazine on May 21, 2020, "Unless we act now to address the mental health needs associated with the pandemic, there will be enormous long-term consequences for families, communities, and societies."

As we have discussed in various parts of this book, nutrition is the foundation of resilience. It cannot remove the stress of any pandemic, but improving our nutrition could facilitate our ability to cope with it. Indeed, there have already been publications showing that people who reported eating more poorly during lockdown also reported deterioration in their mood.[4]

Daily B Complex for Resilience: The Most Overlooked, Inexpensive, and Benign Treatment There Is

Over the last two decades, there has been a considerable body of research in many different countries, including South Africa, the United Kingdom, and Australia, that clearly shows the importance of additional B vitamins as a way to improve resilience in the face of stress. In fact, there are enough studies that if B vitamins were a patentable drug, every physician would probably prescribe them for stress and anxiety! Some of these studies have focused on workplace stress, and others have looked at the effects of these nutrients on university students or healthy individuals in the community. Overall, the research has shown that B vitamins assist with the reduction of general stress, an effect that is observable within a very short period of time.[5]

What this means is that B vitamins can help you cope with all those additional demands that life throws at you, and quickly too. When it became clear that the COVID-19 virus was going to become a pandemic, we encouraged mental health professionals to recommend that their clients try to eat healthy diets, and also take a daily B complex after breakfast to improve their psychological resilience.

Why are B vitamins so important? Because they play a prominent role in the methylation cycle and in making those important neurotransmitters we talked about in the first three chapters. They are also vital for glucose metabolism, which is very important for the fight/flight response as well as for the pathways involved in reducing the effects of inflammation.

What we didn't know until the Christchurch earthquakes in 2010 and 2011 was whether these nutrients could help people overcome the acute and chronic effects of trauma. It took these traumatic earthquakes for proof to emerge.

Nutrients and the Christchurch Earthquakes in 2010 and 2011

Julia: I live in Christchurch, the largest city on the South Island of New Zealand, one of the most scenic places on earth. One reason it has such stunning scenery is because of earthquakes and volcanic activity shaping and carving a landscape of lakes, mountains, and rivers over millions of years. If you live in a seismically active area, you know intellectually that an earthquake could strike at any minute, but this thought is usually pushed to the back of your mind as you go about your life. That strategy was upended when, on September 4, 2010, at 4:35 a.m., a magnitude 7.1 earthquake struck just outside Christchurch.

My husband and I had only been in one earthquake before. We'd been in Mexico, and the quake was as insubstantial as a truck rolling by the hostel we were staying in. The experience on September 4 was a hundred times worse. The noise was relentless and the shaking seemed endless;

it was violent and terrifying. Our thoughts immediately went to our two kids, but the house was shaking so much we had to crawl to their bedrooms. When I reached our youngest, who was six at the time, he said to me: "Mum, am I dead?"

I remember thinking at the time that this earthquake was going to change my life course forever. And it did.

Fortunately, despite enormous destruction of property, no one was killed. And this earthquake provided many different researchers at the University of Canterbury the opportunity to evaluate the before/after effects of this startling and traumatic event. I was running clinical trials using multinutrients to treat ADHD in adults, and happened to be at a stage in my research where some people were taking nutrients (in the form of the EMP formula), and others were not. In the days after the earthquake, the university was closed but we still had to get the pills out to people in our study. A colleague, Professor Emeritus Neville Blampied, and I drove around on broken, cracked roads to deliver them even while aftershocks rocked the city. It was during these travels that I remembered research I had read about as a graduate student that had been done in California to evaluate the effects of an earthquake on an arthritis pain-management program. Once we confirmed that our friends and students were all okay, and that our house was barely damaged despite the shaking, I started thinking about what research we could do in the wake of this disaster — turning such a negative into a positive.

We got quick ethics clearance to contact all current and past participants of our research, and established whether they were taking multinutrients and for how long. We then assessed how anxious, depressed, and stressed these people were one and two weeks post-quake when there were about a thousand aftershocks (as you can see in the figure). We already had data on all of these participants in terms of how they were functioning before the earthquake hit.

The results were illuminating. Although everyone experienced height-

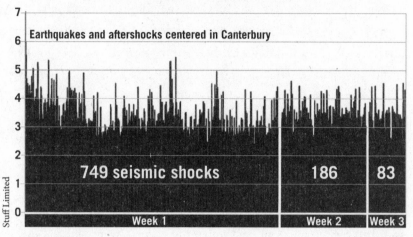

In the Three Weeks Following the Earthquake There Were About 1,000 Aftershocks

Earthquakes and aftershocks centered in Canterbury

749 seismic shocks   186   83

Week 1   Week 2   Week 3

Stuff Limited

ened anxiety and stress just after the event, those who were taking the nutrients at the time of the earthquake recovered more quickly than those who weren't. Two weeks after the earthquake, they were significantly less stressed and anxious than those who weren't taking the pills. The conclusion was that the additional nutrients at the time of extreme stress appeared to assist with buffering the body and mind from the impact of the trauma.[6]

The earthquakes settled down a bit and I returned to my other clinical trials. We were adapting to the new normal, with an aftershock every few hours. Based on the intensity, whether you swayed or rattled, and how long it went on for, we could estimate that earthquake pretty accurately. We played games with our kids — guess that earthquake. Was it a 4.1? 5.3? It was kind of fun in a warped way to take our minds off the fear, and somehow it made it easier to cope. My kids have been remarkably resilient, unlike many other children who are to this day still struggling with severe anxiety because of this prolonged sequence of earthquakes.

A mere five months later, on February 22, 2011, at 12:51 p.m., another major earthquake hit. I was in my office on the fifth floor of the psychology building, getting ready for a conference call. This was not like the previous aftershocks — we were told later that the ground acceleration of that earthquake was the highest ever recorded. You don't really think in those events; you act, doing what needs to be done to survive, just like we discussed earlier in this chapter about the fight/flight response. I dove under my desk and watched my office fall apart: pictures crashing down, books hurtling off the shelves, filing cabinets shaking violently. And the noise. You never forget the noise of an earthquake. When it was over, my colleagues and I evacuated out of the building, not realizing it would be months before we would be allowed back in again.

Afterward, I understood what liquefaction actually was, as so many roads had melted into sand and water. My normal twenty-minute drive home took four hours as I traveled with a university colleague and friend, as well as my former postdoc supervisor, Professors Randy Grace and Rosemary Tannock. Rosemary was visiting on an extended fellowship to our university.

For the entire fraught journey home, I had no contact with my family as I'd left my cellphone in my office, only knowing, based on radio reports, that my suburb was one of the hardest hit. When we finally arrived at our kids' school, I had to brace myself for the worst. The playground had been set up with a sea of tents. There were people everywhere, displaced, lost, shocked. Luckily, I found my family and they were all okay, but my husband broke the news about our home. We couldn't live there. The bricks on the outside of the house had fallen off, the walls were cracked, the hot-water heater on the second floor had broken, and there was water damage everywhere in addition to shattered glass and broken furniture. We slept that night in our garage, wondering how we were going to get through it as aftershock after aftershock rocked the city. It was definitely the worst night of my life.

Although only a magnitude 6.3 quake, this one was much shallower and far more violent and devastating than the previous one. The final death toll was 185 and the central city was destroyed in New Zealand's fifth-deadliest disaster. We all knew someone who had died. For me, it was a former student and colleague, Susan Selway, who was killed when the building she was in collapsed and killed 115 people.

The days following that earthquake were some of the darkest I can recall as we came to grips with the devastating damage to our home and the infrastructure of the city. It was very difficult to work when my office was closed for three months while remedial work was carried out to make it safe to work in, and my husband's workplace was completely destroyed. We were displaced and distraught. There was the constant stress of dealing with insurance issues, and the worries about our children coupled with the guilt that they had to be relocated to a new school and make new friends. I don't know how we would have coped had we not been fortunate enough to move into Rosemary's university-allocated house — where we stayed for 102 days.

It was during this time that I chose to apply what we had learned after the September earthquake and take some extra nutrients to help me cope with the stress. Perhaps they were the reason why I had the mental capacity to come up with the idea of a study on stress, micronutrients, and earthquakes that we could run — even though we had no space, no phones, and virtually no contact with participants.

For three months, my students and I ran clinical trials out of Rosemary's small house. There was a constant stream of people — research assistants, colleagues, students, and research participants — coming and going. By day, the house was a beehive of research and teaching activity; in the evening, there was a beehive of Lego building with our children.

My research team and I designed an online clinical trial where we could compare two different nutrient formulas — Berocca™, a B-complex formula; and EMP, at two different doses. Berocca™ had already been used in three placebo-controlled trials looking at the effects of B vitamins on stress and so we knew it was better than a placebo.[7] EMP was the product we were studying at the time of the September 2010 earthquake, so it made sense to keep using it and to learn about the optimal dose. Ninety-one people were randomized to one of these three treatments (B complex, EMP high dose, EMP low dose). An additional twenty-five people served as a non-randomized control group — we called them a treatment-as-usual condition in that they received the typical care being offered in Christchurch at the time (counseling, medications, or nothing at all). All participants were met in person once to review consent and to give them their nutrients. They were then followed weekly over the internet with questionnaires. The study was completed in three months. We experienced thousands of aftershocks over that short time, indicating that the ongoing stimulation of the fight/flight response continued for all of our participants throughout the trial.

The results were consistent with the study from September. Nutrients helped many people recover from the stress associated with this major natural disaster. The higher dose of EMP (eight capsules/day) had some further advantage in that more people in that group reported greater improvement in mood, anxiety, and energy, with twice as many reporting being "much" to "very much" improved and five times more likely to continue taking EMP post-trial than the Berocca™ group. Those taking the combination of minerals and vitamins (EMP) also reported fewer intrusive thoughts related to the trauma than the Berocca™ group. In addition, for those in any of the three nutrient treatment groups, scores on measures of stress, anxiety, and mood dropped from being in the moderate-severe range down into the normal nonclinical range, but there was very little change for those who received treatment-as-usual. The mean rates of probable post-traumatic stress disorder (PTSD) in the three treated groups dropped from 65 percent to 19 percent. There was no change in the untreated group, with the probable PTSD rates staying at about 50 percent.[8]

The reports from our participants were overwhelmingly positive. One online comment toward the end of the trial was: "I like these pills & believe they have made a huge difference to the way I feel & my perspective of things happening in the city & my life."

These results could have been a result of the placebo effect — which can happen when you simply show compassion and care toward people, and they respond positively. Although this effect could have affected all the groups in our study, it's doubtful that it was the reason for the three nutrient groups to have shown such clear improvement. That's because there are already numerous placebo-controlled studies showing how nutrients are superior to placebo in reducing stress.

Instead, it is more likely that the benefit we observed was due to providing the brain with additional nutrients at a time when supplies were being diverted to the fight/flight response. Remember the Triage Theory? In times of stress, our body's reserves and nutrients are diverted to the fight/flight response, leaving fewer nutritional resources to sustain other normal functions at optimal levels. This can lead to insufficient nutrients for good mental function. Additional nutrients replenish these depleted stores. Maybe that's how we helped so many of those people.

Emily and the Earthquake

When Emily entered our study, she was so shaky and scared, she wouldn't come into the building to meet us—we had to meet her outside on a park bench to discuss the study and what it involved. She had been inside a building in town when the earthquake happened and thought she was going to die when objects started to fall around and on her. She was lucky and ended up with only minor injuries, but she knew many others who had much more severe injuries, and several people she knew lost their lives.

Emily was randomized to receive EMP at the higher dose of four pills twice a day. "The trial really helped me. I honestly felt a big difference within three or four days," she told me. "I felt less tearful and more capable to deal with day-to-day things."

Before taking the multinutrients, she had struggled just to get out of the house, and little things disproportionately irritated her. After the trial, she was taking control of her emotions again and entering buildings without panic. Her scores on our measures of stress and anxiety also reflected the huge change she was noticing.

Emily's story was typical of many of the people who participated in our research in 2011. We kept hearing about how the nutrients were giving the needed boost to help people at a really difficult time in their lives.

Nutrients and the Southern Alberta Flood in 2013

Bonnie: Eighteen months after the second Christchurch earthquake, we had a chance to replicate and extend the research. In June 2013, southern Alberta, Canada, had a very heavy rainfall added to an unusually large amount of snowmelt from the Rocky Mountains, resulting in a catastrophic flood on June 19. I had never been in a disaster of any kind before. And I was fortunate, because I live on a hill, so there was no damage to my home.

Afterward, like many of my fellow citizens, I dug out my tall rubber boots, heavy gloves, a mask, and a shovel. For the next few days I divided my time between the homes of friends who lived right on the river in Calgary, and driving sixty miles south of the city to the town of High River (aptly named for its vulnerability to water events). Each day I would just walk up to a High River home where people were pulling off drywall in an attempt to avoid mold, and I would begin yanking it off the walls and shoveling mud from the basement. To this day, I don't know who I was helping, and they don't know my name either. That's what happens when you have a rare event in an otherwise unstressed population: volunteer help arrives.

Julia, whose in-laws live in Calgary, knew right away what was happening here. She Skyped me and said, "Bonnie, you have to go to your mayor and tell him to distribute nutrients to alleviate PTSD and mental distress!"

Julia's earthquake research was not yet fully published, and it seemed unlikely that our government would be receptive, so she and I decided to do a collaborative study of six weeks of nutrient treatment. We used her online data collection system, which was still available from the earthquake research, and recruited fifty-six adults in Calgary who were suffering from extreme depression, anxiety, and stress following the flood, and who had no prior history of mental disorders. They were randomized to receive a B-vitamin complex (made by Douglas Laboratories), EMP, or 1,000 IU of vitamin D (an active comparator treatment).

Obviously, while difficult and upsetting, a one-day flood in southern Alberta caused nowhere near the magnitude of stress experienced by the citizens of Christchurch, who endured over 8,000 aftershocks in the five months between the two major earthquakes. So we assumed that a nutrient benefit might be difficult to detect after the flood. However, both the B complex and the broad-spectrum multinutrients resulted in significant and much larger improvements in measures of depression, anxiety, and stress compared to the modest improvements following vitamin D.[9] The post-flood results demonstrate the foundational importance of having a well-nourished brain to be resilient to even momentary stresses.

Nutrients and the Fort McMurray Fire in 2016

Bonnie: We both often lecture about these important study results from the earthquakes and the flood. On May 1, 2016, Fort McMurray, a community in northern Alberta, was hit by a devastating wildfire that raged for nearly two months and forced 88,000 people to leave their homes.

At the time of the fire, I suddenly noticed how many adults were wandering around the Calgary area, seemingly with no place to go, and often carrying fast food from the local outlets. I realized that the dorms in the nearby university were housing many of the displaced people. In such a stressful time, these evacuees had to feed their brains whatever they could find — just when they really needed extra minerals and vitamins.

I contacted local authorities, who ignored my pleas to give out information or to provide a B-complex supplement. As a result, from June 2016 to June 2018, physician visits for mood disorders and anxiety disorders increased by almost 50 percent. Even worse is how much the affected children suffered. In 2019, a study from the University of Alberta reported on the very high rate of PTSD in the children who had been displaced by the fire: 37 percent met criteria for probable PTSD; 31 percent for probable depression, 17 percent for probable depression of at least moderate severity; and 27 percent for probable anxiety.[10]

If we had been permitted to provide information about the benefits of supplementary nutrients, we suspect many of those people would not have suffered as they did — and medical expenses would have been greatly reduced for patients and for government-funded treatments.

Nutrients and the Christchurch Mosque Shootings in 2019

Julia: Sadly, we had another opportunity to test the effects of nutrients on stress in Christchurch. On March 15, 2019, during prayers in two different mosques, a white-supremacist terrorist killed fifty-one and injured forty people of the Muslim faith. I knew the psychological recovery would be slow and painful.

Like Bonnie after the Alberta flood, I devoted all my efforts to contacting local authorities — to ensure they were aware that multinutrients were an effective intervention, and urging them to provide them as part of the recovery response. Yet again, they declined to act on this information.[11] This was distressing, as our research indicated that there is a better chance of recovery if nutritional treatment is provided early.

I felt I couldn't stand by and do nothing, given all the data on nutrients and stress, so my lab fundraised to purchase some nutrients (Optimal Balance®) similar to those that had been effective in previous post-disaster research, and we provided them for free to those who self-identified to us from the Muslim community as needing help.

Word of mouth spread through the Muslim community about the nutrients and we gave them to anyone who asked. As responsible clinicians, we monitored the symptoms of those taking the donated nutrients as both an ethical and standard action. We created an online questionnaire as the easiest way to monitor their symptoms over time. We also received further donations from members of the public to support the initiative.

Within weeks, we were clinically monitoring twenty-six people, and, not surprisingly, we saw the exact same treatment effect that we had seen after the earthquakes and the flood. Not everyone got better, but many people did.

Mirwais and the Shooting

Mirwais (he asked that we use his real name) had been at the Al-Noor mosque in Christchurch during the shooting. A bullet had scraped the side of his skull and a few millimeters had been the difference between life and death. Many people died around him that day. When Julia met him, Mirwais had been struggling with depressed mood, fitful sleep, flashbacks, anger, impatience, and fear. He described waking suddenly, sweating, with flashbacks to the event. A couple of hours of sleep was a good night.

Within days of taking the multinutrients, his sleep improved —which is something we often hear, as the nutrients can help sleep get better quite quickly. After a month, Mirwais felt remarkably better. He reported sleeping well without the help of sleeping pills, his mood was more stable, the flashbacks became infrequent, his anger and patience thresholds were back to normal, and he was not afraid anymore. More than a year after the shooting, Mirwais is still doing well and telling his friends and family to take the nutrients. And thanks to continued donations from the community, over a year later, Julia and her team are still giving out the nutrients to anyone in the Muslim community affected by the shootings who asks for them.

Before starting the treatment, 77 percent of those original twenty-six people we monitored met or exceeded a cutoff score defining probable PTSD. After an average of five weeks, this rate dropped to 23 percent. In other words, of all the people who likely had PTSD, 70 percent of them were in remission after about a month of multinutrient treatment.

This was an astonishing finding, and one rarely observed with conventional treatments for PTSD. Mass shootings happen far too often in America, and extreme weather events and natural disasters regularly strike all over the world. All families and victims deserve to know about this simple, affordable intervention. It can reduce stress and mental health

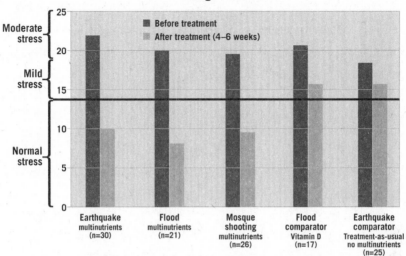

Change in Stress

Below horizontal black line, scores are within normal nonclinical range

issues while improving resilience in the aftermath of a disaster or even an ordinary stressful event.

The bar graph shows that we have established, from three different traumatic events, that broad-spectrum multinutrients are a simple intervention that is easy to track, easy to follow, and *better* than the current standard of care (or lack thereof). We also have government data from the Fort McMurray fire showing what happens when people are *not* offered extra nutrients.

As you learned already, a solution that works so well for people under extreme stress can work for you too, even if your stress is not due to a sudden catastrophe but rather to ongoing issues in your life. There is still lots of research to be done in this space and Julia's lab has a study underway to look at survivors of other traumas, like exposure to domestic violence, rape, and accidents. At this stage, the studies have focused on the beneficial effects of nutrients for acute trauma. We still don't know if nutrients can help with PTSD months or years after the trauma occurred. Hopefully future studies will begin to answer those questions. It will be especially important to determine whether multinutrient treatment could be effectively applied to war veterans or chronic PTSD. We hope one day this information is common knowledge.

The Takeaway

1. The more stressed or traumatized you are, the more you need nutrients to help you cope—and the less likely you are to get them, especially if food supplies are disrupted after a natural disaster, or you understandably turn to comfort foods for temporary relief.

2. After an unexpected trauma, a daily broad-spectrum multinutrient supplement can, after only a few weeks, substantially improve how you're feeling. This is especially worth trying before turning to psychiatric medication. Nutrients may give your brain the additional boost it needs.

3. A vitamin B-complex supplement (taken with food every morning) can improve resilience to trauma and stress, without any side effects except your urine may become a brighter yellow from excess riboflavin being excreted.

4. Multinutrient supplements can also help you manage the normal, everyday stresses of modern life.

Part III

HOW TO FEED YOUR BRAIN

8

FOOD FIRST: EATING WELL, MEDITERRANEAN STYLE

Eat food. Not too much. Mostly plants.

— MICHAEL POLLAN, *In Defense of Food: An Eater's Manifesto*

BEST-SELLING AUTHOR AND JOURNALISM professor Michael Pollan nailed it when he said, "Eat food."

Focus on Real Food First

The best way to eat for optimal brain health is to focus on eating *real food first*. Not the processed chemicals that the food industry refers to as food. If you can follow Pollan's rule, then that is a perfect start on your journey to better mental health.

Focusing on real food isn't about any one prescriptive diet — all you need to do is look at how indigenous people from different countries have thrived on very different diets. What you most need to think about is *variety*, ensuring that your plate contains the colors of the rainbow . . . and that you eat food that our ancestors would recognize as food.

Eating real food means that you stay away from ultra-processed foods. How do you know what they are?

- Ultra-processed foods come in boxes, bags, or cans. They represent two-thirds of all foods sold in supermarkets. They are also found at gas station mini-marts, convenience and dollar stores, and fast food restaurants.
- A long list of ingredients on the label is a primary indicator of an ultra-processed food. If you don't recognize the ingredients (or can't pronounce them), it is almost always an item that has nothing to do with nature!
- These foods are enhanced with food dyes, sodium injections, added sugars, and chemical preservatives.

"Food Matters!"

A comment on Julia's TEDx talk from viewer Sam: "I had been on antidepressants for seven years and tried again and again to get off with no luck until I finally did a massive diet overhaul, got clear about how real nutrition works, and started eating correctly. It's been eight years now since I took my last pill after getting my nutritional routine nailed down PLUS I'm no longer an obese, insomniac binge eater. FOOD MATTERS!!!"

What do we mean by "real food"? The pioneering founder of Integrative Mental Health is Dr. Andrew Weil, the best-selling author, speaker, and founder and director of the Andrew Weil Center for Integrative Medicine at the University of Arizona. This center has been training physicians and allied health providers (from the United States and other countries) for decades about non-pharmaceutical treatments for physical health, and more recently for mental health. Earlier than many medical professionals, Dr. Weil recognized the role of inflammation in mental health disorders. He may have been the first one to use the term "anti-inflammatory diet" to describe the whole-foods-based diet intended to help control the symptoms of excess chronic inflammation, whether the symptoms were caused by a physical ailment like arthritis or a mental health condition like depression. His Anti-Inflammatory Food Pyramid helps with food choices, showing you how to shift your eating to a Mediterranean/Asian dietary pattern. We especially like the term he uses: True Food.

Why is True Food so appealing? Technically, food is defined as something we consume to build and maintain life, such as colorful vegetables, fruits, eggs, fish, meat, and filling whole grains and beans. When you walk down the fresh produce aisles at a supermarket, or go to a farm stand in the summer, think of how good and fresh and enticing everything looks and smells. Then think about how you feel after you've eaten some ultra-processed sugary food: maybe that doughnut or candy bar or bag of potato chips tasted delicious in the moment, but you know you're going to feel leaden and unsatisfied — and hungrier than ever — a short time later when the sugar rush comes and goes.

No ultra-processed food item can come close to giving you the benefits of real food. That's why when we talk about those ultra-processed chemical concoctions as food, we're always tempted to put the word "food" in quotation marks.

Everything that we recommend about healthy eating for optimal mental health focuses on whole food, true food, real food.

How Did Our Grandparents Eat?

Our grandparents and their ancestors consumed fruits and vegetables only in the season in which they grew naturally, which we now know maximizes their nutrient content. They might also have eaten frozen vegetables, which became popular after World War II, and which provided an added benefit of preserving nutrient value better than "fresh" food that may have sat on shelves for a long time. Freezing food in ice cellars is actually an ancient practice, but it was not until 1927 that a man named Clarence Birdseye applied for a patent for a system of freezing food. Little did he know how his brilliant idea would, decades later, morph into microwavable meatball "sandwiches" unlike any real food our ancestors would recognize!

The process of canning had been invented over a century prior to that, but canning food was driven primarily by the need to preserve foods carried by soldiers; initially, canned food was not seen as a staple of the family diet. (An oddity associated with this fact is that the can *opener* was not invented until 1858, about fifty years after the invention of the can. There was no need, because soldiers used their bayonets to open their food cans. When the Napoleonic wars ended, canned food spread to home use, and bayonets no longer offered an ideal solution for the average household!)

By the mid-twentieth century, it was generally thought that frozen and canned food had become a huge boon to nutrient intake in North America, as they diversified the average family's diet. It is important to remember that fact, as the term "processed food" is now more commonly thought of as a negative thing, but a hundred years ago "processed" meant canned or frozen — two inventions that likely improved many people's vegetable intake. So unless you pluck apples directly off a tree or drink milk straight from a cow, the vast majority of foods we eat are technically processed. This doesn't necessarily make them "unhealthy." A can of diced tomatoes, for example, that contains only tomatoes and a tiny bit of salt or citric acid as preservatives is not unhealthy. Ditto for cans or frozen bags of beans or other vegetables or fruits that have few added ingredients.

Another difference in how our grandparents thought about food is that most of them would have been unfamiliar with the idea of food *advertising,* and especially advertising directed at children. Children were expected to eat whatever the adults prepared. And in many middle-class families, the moms were likely at home full-time, and responsible for all the food shopping and cooking. Long hours of shopping and preparation were typically required because the food items were fresh, and as yet unavailable in ready-to-cook packages. They bought their food from neighborhood shops and butchers, and they also grew some of their produce and bought some directly from farmers.

The Foods That Give You the Essential Brain-Health Nutrients You Need

In a 2018 article for the *World Journal of Psychiatry*, psychiatrists Laura LaChance and Drew Ramsey published a novel analysis of foods, based on their nutrient profiles, that would be best as "anti-depressant foods."[1] This is the first attempt that we're aware of that carefully connected the research on specific nutrients with foods rich in those nutrients. On the list were vitamins such as folate, thiamine, vitamin A, vitamin B6, vitamin B12, and vitamin C; minerals such as iron, magnesium, potassium, selenium, and zinc; and omega-3 fatty acids (EPA and DHA). The one drawback to their summary was that the studies they drew from were mostly single-nutrient studies, which we have highlighted as having limitations, but it was the closest analysis to date that identified the foods containing the nutrients known to be important for reducing depression.

What did Drs. LaChance and Ramsey find to be our top brain foods? For animal foods, the highest scores were for bivalves such as oysters and mussels, other seafood, and organ meats. For plant foods, the highest scores were for leafy greens, lettuces, peppers, and cruciferous vegetables — such as broccoli, kale, and cauliflower. All of these foods are an integral part of the Mediterranean diet.

It's unfortunate that we need to strike a word of caution for those who like to eat oysters and mussels, but it's important to know where they are gathered. Bivalves struggle to eliminate toxins from their environment; in polluted waters, things like marine algal toxins can accumulate, which would outweigh any health benefits.[2] So be careful!

The Nutrient List for Mental Health

As mentioned, the novel approach to mental health nutrients reported by Drs. LaChance and Ramsey was limited by the single-nutrient studies on which it was based. In reality, the list of nutrients known to contribute to brain function is much longer, but easy to summarize by category:

- All the minerals needed by our soil to be healthy — there are about fifteen: Boron, calcium, chromium, copper, iodine, iron, lithium, magnesium, manganese, molybdenum, phosphorus, potassium, selenium, vanadium, zinc
- All the vitamins produced by crops grown in that soil — also about fifteen: Vitamins A, B1 through 12, C, D, E, and K
- The essential fatty acids: Particularly omega-3s
- All the phytonutrients that healthy plants package along with the above: Currently estimated to be approximately 10,000! Since most are not yet defined or studied, this is the best argument of all for eating lots of whole foods made from plants.
- All the proteins and amino acids produced by healthy crops — there are about twenty-two essential amino acids

So what are we supposed to do with that knowledge? After all, when we look at something like an eggplant in the grocery store, we currently have no way to analyze what nutrients it actually contains. (Although people are working on handheld meters to do exactly that, as mentioned in chapter 3). Even if we are buying food in packages, we are not about to memorize all the nutrient names and carry a list to examine their labels. And manufacturers never include the trace minerals such as molybdenum on their labels — have you ever even heard of that one? How will we know what to buy?

You don't need to learn biochemistry to do your grocery shopping!

That is why we are not specifying lists and lists of nutrients, or explaining that lithium is in this vegetable but not that one. Our goal is to *help* people with mental health challenges, not to make everything more confusing! The solution really is simple:

- Buy real food, true food; avoid ultra-processed food.
- Include slightly processed foods (like canned and frozen items) that do not have a lot of added sugar and preservatives if these items make your cooking easier.
- Always try to change things up and increase your variety. Look for new things to add to your menu as often as possible. Strive to do so every week. What if you don't know how to eat purple-topped turnips? This week read up on them, and you'll see that they're great raw, sliced and put into salads, or dipped into hummus.
- Try an easy new recipe each week, and ask your family members to keep you company (and help out!) in the kitchen.
- Remember that dark, leafy greens are a great source of some of those B vitamins you need for resilience, though B12 is best obtained from animal protein.
- Meat, fish, and eggs are good sources of protein, helping to regulate blood sugar and appetite as well as providing bioavailable iron and zinc.

You are now on your way to eating a whole foods, true foods, real foods, Mediterranean type of diet. Use whatever label you prefer — just take that first step toward feeding your brain what it needs.

Mediterranean and Traditional Diets Are Best for Optimal Mental Health

There are many healthy ways to eat, but the many years of research we reviewed in chapter 4 showed that the diet with the most beneficial effects for mental health is the Mediterranean type of diet. All the practical details can be found in this chapter.

Think of your diet like two sides of a coin: you can focus on the things that you should *not* eat, and you can focus on the things that you should eat *more* of. The Mediterranean style of eating focuses on the positive, helping you to eat more of the healthy food. The Mediterranean diet is simple, old-fashioned, and closest to what your grandparents probably ate. It includes fresh foods, and is high in vegetables and fruits, nuts, healthy fats, dairy products, lean meat, fish, and whole grains. It's low in — you guessed it! — processed packaged foods.

Traditional diets are comprised primarily of locally grown food. The traditional diet of the Inuit people of far northern climates is very different from the traditional diet of Māori (the indigenous people of New Zealand), but the locals each thrive on those foods. The Inuit have greater access to seal, for example, whereas Māori have greater access to eel, fish, and berries. One of the terrible effects of migration and colonization has been the removal of traditional foods from everyday diets.

What About Other Popular Diet Trends?

Many of the popular diets focus on eating whole, true foods. But they also tend to be highly restrictive, making them a bit difficult to sustain.

Gluten-Free and/or Casein-Free Diet (GFCF)

Gluten-free is now a "trendy" way to eat, but one of its big problems is that most people self-diagnose with little understanding of gluten, gain weight, pay extra for gluten-free items, then give up. In fact, the comedian Jimmy Kimmel did a segment on his show where people who claimed to be gluten-free were asked what gluten was — and none of them knew that it's a protein found in grains like wheat, rye, spelt, and barley!

Most gluten-free processed foods are high in fat and sugar, making them calorie-dense, and high in preservatives and color additives. Wheat flour is usually replaced with rice flour, which is also processed and nutrient-poor; and, unless carefully monitored, fiber consumption declines when whole grains are avoided. For those with celiac disease or true sensitivity, however, a gluten-free diet can be a lifesaver.

If you have a child with autism, you've likely heard about the GFCF diet. It removes all sources of gluten as well as casein, a protein found in milk, from the diet. Some scientists believe that these proteins can cause digestive issues in people sensitive to them, which can then lead to suboptimal brain functioning.

There are countless anecdotal reports of positive behavioral effects from eliminating these two proteins. This is not surprising, given that there are often digestive issues associated with autism. The challenge is determining whether these children got better because they stopped eating gluten and casein, or because their diet improved when it was changed. Were processed and sweet foods replaced with more vegetables?

Some studies have confirmed parental observations about their children getting better,[3] whereas others concluded that there wasn't enough evidence to support GFCF diets for ASD.[4] There might be a subset of individuals for whom GFCF does help. One study that only included kids with digestive issues showed that a GFCF diet helped both gut issues and ASD symptoms.[5]

In addition, there is significant clinical evidence showing that casein and gluten sensitivity can exist in some people with mood disorders and schizophrenia.[6] People with celiac disease are at greater risk of having psychiatric problems, either because of their restricted diet and/or because the diet can cause gut problems — which, as you learned in chapter 3, can then lead to negative effects on brain function.

Given that the evidence isn't definitive, you might try a GFCF diet for a few weeks or months and see how you feel. Ask your physician whether there are useful tests for these sensitivities. Then you may want to work with a credentialed nutritionist to ensure you don't inadvertently cause nutritional deficiencies. Be mindful when buying gluten-free products, as they can contain ingredients your gut and brain may not appreciate.

A1 or A2 Milk?

One reason why getting rid of casein in milk may help or resolve some symptoms might be due to what *type* it is. Most people don't know that there are actually two types of casein: A1 and A2.

Most of the dairy cows in the Western world (Europe, North America, New Zealand) are the A1 variant. Parts of Asia and Africa seem to have primarily A2 dairy cows. A1 casein may be associated with a range of human health issues due to the effect of BCM7 — a small piece of protein, called a peptide, which is released by A1 casein — getting through leaky guts and affecting the brain. People with ASD/schizophrenia have been found to excrete large quantities of BCM7 in their urine, and it's been thought that their symptoms may be exacerbated by A1 milk but reversed if they switch to A2 milk.[7] If given the choice, and especially if you are suffering from dairy intolerance, it's worth seeing if A2 milk will make a difference. Products like cheese that contain or have used A2 milk will make it clear on the label. It's harder to find and more expensive, but ask at your local health food stores. Or, you might want to try alternatives like oat or almond "milk"; we aren't aware of any mental health benefits or adverse effects from those products.

Vegetarian and Vegan Diets

There are many different types of vegetarians. A vegan diet is exclusively plant-based, with no consumption of any animal products, not even dairy and eggs. These diets have become increasingly popular, not just for health reasons but because many believe they may create a lower carbon footprint than an omnivore diet.

But are they good for mental health? The evidence is still mixed. Some studies show the vegetarian diet is associated with lowered rates of anxiety and depression,[8] while others show elevated risk.[9] In some studies, *higher* rates of mood and anxiety disorders were found among vegetarians compared to matched non-vegetarians, at twelve months and lifetime prevalence.

There are population-based studies indicating that a small amount of meat is good for your mental health, associated with half the rate of depression.[10] Given that it's an excellent source of some key nutrients, like B12 and iron, these results aren't surprising.

At this point, we can't advocate for an exclusively plant-based diet for optimal mental health, knowing that the scientific results have been inconsistent. But many people seem to thrive on plant-based diets, given their large intake of minerals and vitamins from all that produce, but they do typically add iron, zinc, and vitamin B12 supplements to compensate for the absence of animal protein.

Supplementation may be necessary for some vegetarians and vegans. We are concerned about a vegan diet during pregnancy, knowing how important omega-3s (especially EPA and DHA) are for fetal brain development, although expectant mothers who get all the nutrients they need, in food and possibly with additional supplementation, should be fine.[11] While there are vegan sources of EFAs (such as seeds, nuts, flax, chia, walnuts, and hemp seeds), these EFAs are usually in the form of alpha-linolenic acid, which is poorly converted to EPA and DHA. (Estimates are that just 5 to 10 percent of ALA from flax, for example, is converted to EPA and 2 to 5 percent to DHA.) In other words, 90 percent of plant-based sources of omega-3s are not giving vegans the essential fatty acids their brains may need. Remember, the mental health benefits come from EPA and DHA, not ALA.

For vegans, a better source of EPA and DHA is seaweed or algae, depending on the type. A three-ounce serving of seaweed provides about 100 mg of EPA, but little DHA. In contrast, three ounces of salmon delivers about 1,500 mg EPA+DHA. So to get the same amount of EPA+DHA from seaweed, you would have to eat a whopping 45 ounces — that's nearly three pounds. That's a *lot* of seaweed!

Vegetarians and vegans also need to be concerned about vitamin B12 deficiency, as B12 is essential for the proper development and functioning of brain and nerve cells, and also plays an important role in the synthesis of fatty acids contained in the myelin sheath that surrounds and protects nerves. Because B12 is best sourced from meat, eggs, fish, and dairy, vegetarians/vegans are at greater risk for a B12 deficiency than omnivores.[12] All vegetarians/vegans should consider regular B12 supplementation as well as iron, which is more bioavailable when consumed from animal protein.

The Keto Diet

Originally explored for intractable epileptic seizures, the ketogenic (keto) diet has become extremely popular, mostly because it can lead to rapid weight loss. It's a high-fat, high-protein, low-carbohydrate diet that forces the brain to use ketones, chemicals produced in the liver, to burn fat when your body doesn't have enough glucose as its main source of energy. Because fat is burned, weight comes off.

Most of the research on brain health has focused on keto's potential role in the prevention of Alzheimer's disease. Any diet that is designed to regulate glucose should result in cognitive benefits. One key factor is that keto reduces inflammation. Neurologist Dale Bredesen, a professor at the University of California, Los Angeles, has popularized the keto diet, although his book title, *The End of Alzheimer's: The First Program to Prevent and Reverse the Cognitive Decline of Dementia,* is probably a bit exaggerated, as no controlled studies have been done to date using the keto diet as a prevention tool for Alzheimer's.

Although some studies have shown promising antidepressant and mood-stabilizing effects of keto,[13] research on its beneficial effects on *mental health* is very preliminary, so we can't recommend it as a diet that might help with psychiatric symptoms.

Paleo, GAPS, Wahls, FODMAP, Intermittent Fasting, and Personalized Foods

Several other diets focus on whole foods, and on improving the gut microbiome. One example is the Paleo diet, which guides you to eat only what our ancestors ate during the Paleolithic Age. Another is the Gut and Psychology Syndrome (GAPS) designed by Dr. Natasha Campbell-McBride, a British-based physician, which is quite strict in its early phases (no grains, dairy, starchy vegetables, or refined carbohydrates), though during maintenance it strongly resembles the Mediterranean diet, with the added daily requirement of bone broth and fermented foods. Also similar is the Wahls diet created by Dr. Terry Wahls, an American physician diagnosed with multiple sclerosis. Many people believe that her recommendations have helped their brains to function better, even after a serious brain injury.[14] Like the GAPS diet it features whole foods, lots of fruits and vegetables, healthy oils, nuts, and seeds, plus lots of bone broth and fermented foods. The FODMAP diet (Fermentable Oligosaccharides, Disaccharides, Monosaccharides, and Polyols) is another example, often recommended for those with chronic gut issues.

Intermittent fasting helps with weight loss, improves energy, and may provide clearer thinking. One of the common methods (called 16/8) is to restrict eating to zero calories for sixteen hours, then consume all your meals within an eight-hour period.

Finally, there is a growing focus on using genetics to determine what foods might be right for you. However, we don't think there is any scientific evidence yet that this "personalized" approach is useful for optimizing your mental health. Those studies simply don't exist. If you follow the steps outlined in the next chapter, you really shouldn't need to get your genetic and biomarker profiles done.

What do all these diets have in common? There isn't enough scientific evidence for any of them in terms of mental health benefits, which is why we touch on them so briefly. But they focus on whole foods, avoiding processed foods, and improving gut function. Their restrictiveness, however, can make them hard to stick to in the long term. And that is why we recommend that you *begin* with a Mediterranean-style diet, which you'll find later in this chapter. Tweaking things later — to avoid grains, to cut down on dairy, or to include fermented foods — may also be worth a try as a second step.

Does Skipping Breakfast Affect Your Mental Health?

In the past few decades, there have been dozens of studies looking at overall breakfast habits.

Most of the research looked at what *time* breakfast was eaten, but not so much at *what* was eaten. Some research with adolescents reported on the glycemic index (GI), which shows how quickly blood glucose levels rise after you eat a specific food, relative to the consumption of glucose itself, which is set at a GI of 100. So, for example, a simple carbohydrate like a piece of white toast will cause blood glucose to rise quickly, which is why white bread has a high GI of 75. In one study, adolescents who habitually skipped breakfast were evaluated with cognitive tasks before and after eating a low-GI breakfast, as well as before and after a few hours in the morning when they didn't eat any breakfast.[15] The low-GI breakfast was associated with better subjective reports of alertness and contentment, as well as generally better performance on word recall and other tasks. Other studies have shown that the low-GI breakfast tended to give participants improved performance on learning and memory tasks. In addition, many larger studies have shown that regularly eating breakfast was consistently associated with better academic performance.[16]

The message is clear: If you want to be at your sharpest in the morning and improve mood and stress, eat a good-quality breakfast.[17] To be as sharp as possible, eat a low-GI breakfast!

If you're wondering what an ideal breakfast might be, first make sure that you and your children *eat something* before running off to school and work. Since the morning meal has to sustain a child for several hours of academic instruction, a low-GI breakfast, containing protein and complex carbohydrates, is most likely to help them concentrate. Try a vegetable omelet, plain unsweetened Greek yogurt with fresh strawberries, apple slices with peanut butter, scrambled eggs with avocado and toasted sesame seeds, cottage cheese with fruit and nuts, or steel-cut oatmeal with milk.

Eating Well, Mediterranean Style

Why is a whole foods, Mediterranean-style diet so good for you? One of the reasons is that by eating lots of fresh fruits and vegetables every day, you're not only optimizing your chances of getting a full spectrum of minerals and vitamins — you're also getting them in balance. Real food provides nutrients in the most brilliant combinations, and whole foods contain hundreds or thousands of bioactive phytonutrients, or plant-based chemicals, that provide the rich colors: the reds of apples and watermelon, the dark greens of leafy vegetables and avocado, the yellows/

oranges of citrus fruit and sweet potatoes, and the blues/purples of berries and plums.

Phytonutrients can only be found in whole, real foods. Scientists have already identified several hundred of them — you may have heard of the resveratrol in red wine, the lycopene in tomatoes, or the sulfides in onions and garlic. Most of them don't have names yet, and very few have defined functions. Since we don't yet know what these thousands of phytonutrients actually do, they can't be classified as "essential" nutrients — but we think it's fair to assume that they do confer some health benefits. But you get them only when you eat whole, real foods — where they occur together in the proper balance. They are not in processed food, and few are available (or recommended) as supplements.

Does eating a whole-food-based diet mean you should never have a piece of candy again? Or a croissant? Or chocolate cake? Or French fries? Of course not. We need to feed our brains, but we need to enjoy life, too! Some people follow the 80/20 rule: If you eat healthy whole foods 80 percent of the time, then you can still occasionally enjoy some homemade baked goods or store-bought processed foods for their flavor without worrying about their nutrient density.

And when you do eat those foods, savor every morsel. Telling yourself you're "cheating" or "bad" is a guaranteed recipe for more "cheating."

Eating the Mediterranean way is very simple. Americans usually think of vegetables and carbs as side dishes, but now you're going to flip that and have the veggies be the main dish, followed by the carbs and the protein. The easiest way to do this is to divide your plate into quarters, such as the one shown for the Healthy Eating Plate developed at Harvard School of Public Health. Half the plate should be veggies and some fruit. One-quarter should be whole grains, and one-quarter should be protein and fats.

These tips shown in the figure come from the Australian group that studied the Modified Mediterranean (ModiMed) diet described in chapter 4.[18]

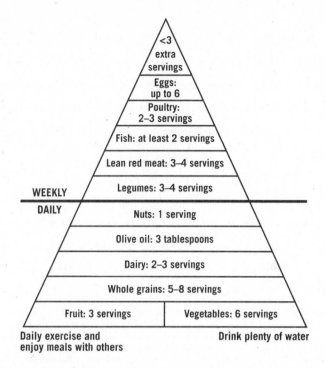

WEEKLY

<3 extra servings

Eggs: up to 6

Poultry: 2–3 servings

Fish: at least 2 servings

Lean red meat: 3–4 servings

Legumes: 3–4 servings

DAILY

Nuts: 1 serving

Olive oil: 3 tablespoons

Dairy: 2–3 servings

Whole grains: 5–8 servings

Fruit: 3 servings   Vegetables: 6 servings

Daily exercise and   Drink plenty of water
enjoy meals with others

From *Nutritional Neuroscience* 21, Issue 7, by permission of Taylor & Francis Ltd.

How a Whole Food Diet Can Make You Feel

A comment from TEDx viewer Stewart: "I switched to a whole food diet for health problems and was amazed at how it has affected my mood. For the first time in eight years, I made it through an entire day without a single panic attack or depressive episode."

Eating Well on a Budget

Eating well doesn't have to be expensive. In one of the Australian studies we told you about in chapter 4, a cost analysis for twenty of the participants showed that their pre-treatment food was costing them (in Australian dollars) an average of $138 per week, which dropped to $112 per week after they learned how to eat the healthier Mod*i*Med diet.[19]

Does this surprise you? People often assume they can't afford healthy fresh food, but they sometimes overlook the fact that processed, packaged, ready-to-eat food, as well as what you can buy in a fast food restaurant, is usually more expensive. Unless you plan to eat lobster and steak every week, home-cooked healthy food will save you money. Here are our favorite tips:

- Cook at home! Restaurant food, whether it's from a fast food, ethnic, or high-end restaurant, is going to be more expensive than a healthy meal you make yourself. If cooking is really new to you, begin by cooking at least once a week and then increase from there.
- If you're a newbie cook, or if you simply want an easier approach (and money is not too big a concern), explore meal delivery kits from companies such as Home Chef, Blue Apron, Sun Basket, Imperfect Food, or HelloFresh. Look for one with minimal packaging to reduce your environmental footprint. You'll be delighted to learn lots of good recipes based on fresh, whole foods.
- Always have staples in your pantry (see shopping list in the next section). Buying larger amounts of items like rice or dried beans, *if you will use them*, can really help — a 6.4 ounce box of a popular rice side dish can, for example, cost as much as a three-pound bag of rice!
- Buy fresh produce in season and look for specials. Consider local farmers' markets. Have fun talking to the farmers — they really know a lot about their crops.
- Every time you cook at home, make at least one extra portion to eat as leftovers the next day, to take to work/school for lunch, or to freeze for future meals.
- Spend a few minutes each week planning meals and making a grocery list. There are many different apps, such as Mealtime, Plan to Eat, Make My Plate, and Eat This Much, that make this easier than you think.

- Never go food shopping when you're hungry! Also, never go food shopping without a list — and stick to it.
- The outer aisles of the supermarket are where the whole foods are found. It's tempting to get sucked into the center aisles and be lulled into buying the latest specials (likely ultra-processed foods), but for the most part, you'll probably regret it.
- Be aware of supermarket tricks to entice you into buying more-expensive food items. For example, more-expensive products tend to be shelved at eye level, and cheaper items are placed on either the upper or lower shelves.
- Shopping and cooking with a friend or relative could help share expenses, provide support and skills, and exchange knowledge. It's also a great way to spend time with your children. The more time they spend with you in the kitchen, the more they'll learn about real food and how to cook it.
- Look for special local programs, like communal vegetable gardens. You might find community kitchens, soup kitchens, produce delivery options, or a nationwide program like Wholesome Wave (which you can read about in chapter 12).

The Mediterranean Diet Shopping List

Before you go food shopping, we recommend a pantry purge of all the unhealthy foods you're no longer going to want. Go through every shelf. Next, do the same for items in your freezer.

Now it's time to go shopping. Below is a list of things that might be useful to have on hand, but your own personal preferences and tastes will influence which ones you buy. Don't feel like you need to go out and buy all of these at once, but over time, your pantry will be transformed and you'll just need to replenish your regular staples. You may also need some other ingredients for the Better Brain Recipes in chapter 9.

Canned, Bottled, or Boxed Goods

Assorted canned fruits and vegetables that you like

Canned fish that you like (e.g., salmon, sardines, tuna)

Chicken or vegetable broth

Coconut milk

Pasta sauce (without sugar added), though it's better if you make your own

Tomatoes, canned, jarred, or boxed; whole, crushed, diced, or pureed;
    tomato sauce; tomato paste

Dry Goods

Dried beans, chickpeas, lentils, and peas

Grains that you like: bulgur, cornmeal, couscous, farro, quinoa,
    wheat berries

Nuts and nut butter: almond, cashew, peanut

Pasta, preferably whole grain

Oats, steel-cut or regular (avoid sweetened instant oatmeal in packets,
    which is highly processed)

Rice, preferably brown

Seeds: chia, pumpkin, sesame, sunflower

Oils and Condiments

Mustard, Dijon mustard

Olive oil: extra virgin (for salads); regular blended olive oil (for cooking);
    avocado oil, coconut oil, sesame oil (for salads and cooking)

Spices and herbs: salt and ground pepper; basil, chives, cilantro, coriander,
    cumin, mint, oregano, paprika, thyme

Vinegar

Fresh Food

Bread, whole grain

Cheese

Chicken breasts, skinless

Eggs

Fish

Fresh fruits and veggies

Milk, dairy or other

Red meats that you like

Tofu: firm for stir-fries; tempeh

Yogurt, plain or Greek (unsweetened)

Basic Kitchen Tools

The basics you need: A few good knives, measuring cups and spoons, non-wooden cutting boards, glass containers for micro-waving/food storage, and non-stick pots and pans.

These four additional tools will enable you to increase your repertoire (without increasing your time in the kitchen) of low-cost, whole foods meals:

- An Instant Pot is basically a high-tech pressure cooker that cooks one-pot meals much more quickly than a stovetop or oven. It's ideal for cooking dried beans and whole grains, and for making yogurt or bone broth. It can also be a slow cooker.
- An air fryer or convection oven can also speed up cooking time. An air fryer is ideal for those who really like fried food, as its dry heat allows you to fake-fry veggies and chicken without added oil.
- An immersion blender is handy for pureeing soups or stews.
- A food processor makes chopping vegetables a breeze.

The Takeaway

1. The Mediterranean, whole food type of diet is best overall to give your brain the nutrients it needs. Beginning with it is a smart way to go. As a second step later on, you may want to try one of the more restrictive diets—such as Paleo or keto—though they haven't yet been proven to improve mental health. Eating diets traditional to your culture and community may also give you helpful nutrients.

2. We suggest a variety of fruits and veggies every day; lots of beans and legumes; at least two servings per week of fish; whole grains; healthy oils; meat and dairy. And you will be amazed at how much money you will save if you have been eating either restaurant food or highly processed items.

3. Always consider leftovers from the previous dinner as your go-to lunch.

4. And finally—what about desserts? There are several in chapter 9. We think you'll know how to find sweet things! Avoid processed baked goods, and explore dark chocolate, fresh or dried fruit, Greek yogurt with honey, or homemade whipped cream over berries.

9

THE BETTER BRAIN RECIPES

IF YOU WANT TO save a lot of money on food and improve your nutrient intake at the same time, these recipes are ideal. We worked with award-winning cookbook author Judith Choate to create them, following the general guidelines of the Mediterranean diet. We think you will find them not only easy to make, but incredibly delicious and satisfying. We included some of our favorite recipes in this section, too, like our go-to granola recipes, Bonnie's favorite mid-morning snack, and Julia's easy, portable lunch recipe.

Fresh, filling, and just what your brain needs. You will notice that one of the things we focus on is adding a lot of legumes to your meals — beans, lentils, and chickpeas. We certainly don't expect you to eat them every day, but they are economical powerhouses of nutrients and fiber, so you'll want to use them in your cooking as often as possible. Lentils cook so fast that it is usually pointless to buy them in cans. And chickpeas are also pretty fast. But dried white beans, kidney beans, and black beans require this process: rinse and put them in fresh water to soak (at least two inches of water above the beans) for eight hours or, even better, overnight; then rinse again and simmer them in fresh water (again, two inches above the beans) for several hours. If using dried beans, use the 2:1 conversion rate; if your recipe calls for 1 cup of cooked beans, soak and cook ½ cup of dried beans. You will have a little left over, and they are great in your salads (especially chickpeas!). *Alternatively,* use an Instant Pot or buy them in cans. Buying beans in cans is a very reasonable choice: still cheap, and they are fully cooked and ready to eat. Just be aware that most have sodium added, so drain them when you open the can or (if you want to get rid of even more of the salt) drain and rinse them.

Breakfast

Bonnie's Classic Granola

    4 cups rolled oats
    1 cup pumpkin seeds
    1 cup sunflower seeds
    1 cup sliced or chopped almonds, or other nuts like walnuts,
        pecans, or Brazil
    1 cup coconut flakes
    1 teaspoon ground cinnamon
    ⅜ cup avocado or canola oil
    ⅛ cup honey

JULIA'S SUGGESTIONS FOR ADDITIONAL SWEETNESS
    ½ cup dried fruit
    ¼ cup dark chocolate chips

Preheat oven to 325°F.

Use parchment paper to line a baking sheet with sides.

In a large bowl, mix together all the dry ingredients.

In a smaller bowl or big measuring cup, mix together oil and honey, and add ¼ cup of water. Heat in microwave for 20 seconds or so — this thins it for easy mixing.

Pour wet mixture over dry ingredients, then mix until oats are moistened. Spread on baking sheet.

Cook for 20 minutes, then stir a little; then return to oven for another 15 minutes.

Cool completely and then stir in the dried fruit and chocolate chips if you are using them. Store in an airtight container. Enjoy in milk or in plain unsweetened yogurt, with fresh berries on top.

Beautiful Green Frittata

SERVES 4

This is such a pretty frittata, filled with healthy protein and greens. It's great for breakfast, but could be a satisfying lunch or dinner also.

6 large eggs, beaten, at room temperature

¾ cup ricotta cheese, well drained

Salt and pepper

1 tablespoon olive oil

1 small onion, peeled and finely chopped

¼ cup chopped chives

½ teaspoon minced garlic

2 cups chopped fresh asparagus

2 cups chopped fresh spinach

Preheat the oven to 350°F.

Combine the eggs with the cheese in a large mixing bowl, whisking to combine. Season with salt and pepper.

Heat the oil in a medium frying pan over medium heat. Add the onion, chives, and garlic and cook, stirring frequently, for about 3 minutes or just until softened. Stir in the asparagus and spinach.

When combined, scrape the vegetable mixture into the eggs. Season with salt and pepper. Pour into a large nonstick, ovenproof skillet, taking care that the vegetables are evenly distributed.

Transfer to the preheated oven and bake uncovered for about 20 minutes or until the frittata is set in the center and the bottom is golden brown.

Remove from the oven and let rest for 5 minutes.

Cut into wedges and serve with a tossed salad or sliced tomatoes on the side, if desired.

Note: You can add some things to make this lovely frittata fit your own tastes. Add hot sauce, serve with parmesan cheese to sprinkle over it, or have some salsa on the side. Also, consider the Stuffed Sweet Potatoes (page 216) as a perfect side dish.

Soups

Easy Leek and Pea Soup

SERVES 4

This is the quickest, easiest, and most delicious soup.

    2 teaspoons olive oil

    1 teaspoon unsalted butter

    3 large leeks, white part only, well washed and chopped

    4 cups low-sodium chicken or vegetable broth

    One 12-ounce package frozen peas

    2 tablespoons chopped fresh mint leaves or ¼ teaspoon dried
        mint

    Sea salt and pepper

    ¼ cup sour cream or plain yogurt, optional

Heat the oil and butter in a medium saucepan over medium heat. Add leeks and cook, stirring frequently, for about 5 minutes or until they begin to soften.

Add the broth and peas and bring to a simmer. Season with salt and pepper, cover, lower the heat, and cook at a gentle simmer for about 10 more minutes or until the vegetables are tender.

Remove from the heat and process to a smooth puree using either a hand-held immersion blender or a standard blender.

Taste and, if necessary, season with additional salt and pepper.

Stir in the mint and place an equal portion into each of four shallow soup bowls. Serve with a dollop of sour cream or plain yogurt in the center.

Thai Green Curry Soup

SERVES 4 TO 6

You won't believe how the ginger and spices wake up your taste buds, and this soup is full of anti-inflammatory spices and healthy vegetables.

2 teaspoons coconut oil

1 tablespoon minced ginger

1 teaspoon minced garlic

1 teaspoon minced green chile (from 1–2 chiles) or to taste

3 tablespoons green curry paste, such as Thai Kitchen

One 13.5-ounce can coconut milk

3 cups water

Sea salt and cracked black pepper

2 cups (about 1 pound) chopped broccoli florets

2 cups spinach leaves

1 cup chopped cilantro (leaves and stems)

Sliced scallions, mint, or cilantro leaves for serving, optional

Place oil in a large saucepan over medium heat. Add ginger, garlic, and chile and cook, stirring occasionally, for 3 minutes. Stir in the curry paste and cook for an additional minute.

Add coconut milk along with 3 cups of cold water. Season with salt and pepper and bring to a simmer.

Add the broccoli, cover, and bring to a simmer. Cook, covered, for about 12 minutes or until the broccoli is tender.

Remove from heat and add the spinach and cilantro. Using a hand-held immersion blender (or a high-speed stand-alone blender), process to a smooth puree.

Taste and, if necessary, season with salt and pepper.

Serve, garnished with scallions, mint, or cilantro, if desired.

Minestrone Soup for Instant Pot or Stovetop

SERVES 4 TO 6

If you use the dried and canned ingredients specified, you will end up with an incredibly inexpensive and healthy minestrone soup that will probably last you two to three days.

> 2 tablespoons olive oil
>
> 1 large red onion, peeled and diced
>
> 1 teaspoon minced garlic
>
> 2 stalks celery, trimmed and diced
>
> 2 medium carrots, peeled, trimmed, and diced
>
> 1 teaspoon dried oregano
>
> 1 teaspoon dried basil
>
> ½ teaspoon dried thyme
>
> 1 tablespoon tomato paste
>
> Salt and pepper
>
> One 28-ounce can diced tomatoes with their juice
>
> 2 medium zucchini, trimmed and diced
>
> 1 cup dried cannellini or other white beans, rinsed
>   (see Note)
>
> 1 cup dried small soup pasta such as orzo or ditalini or other
>   small dried pasta
>
> 6 cups low-sodium vegetable broth or water
>
> 3 cups chopped greens such as spinach, Swiss chard, or kale,
>   optional

2 tablespoons chile garlic sauce or other preferred hot sauce,
     optional

Parmesan cheese for serving, optional

Place the oil in the Instant Pot and press the Sauté button to heat it for a minute or so. Add onions and garlic. Cook, stirring occasionally, for about 3 minutes or until starting to soften and become very aromatic.

Add the celery, carrots, oregano, basil, and thyme, stirring to lightly coat with the oil. Add the tomato paste, season with salt and pepper, and cook, stirring for another 3 minutes.

Add the tomatoes, zucchini, beans, and pasta along with the broth and just enough water to cover the mixture by about 1 inch. Mix well.

Press Cancel and close the lid. Pressure cook (high) on Manual for 40 minutes. Carefully do a Quick Release.

Add the greens, taste, and, if necessary, season with salt and pepper. Allow the soup to sit for a few minutes to allow the greens to soften.

If you like spice, add your favorite hot sauce.

Serve piping hot with a sprinkling of Parmesan cheese, if desired.

Note: This can be easily made on a stovetop with a large soup pot. Use cooked beans that you have prepared ahead of time from dried beans (see directions on page 201) or use canned beans, added at the same point as the dried beans in the above recipe. The stovetop cook time will be about 45 minutes or until the soup has thickened and the flavors have blended. It's fine for the vegetables to be very soft.

Ginger-Parsnip Soup

SERVES 4 TO 6

We love this unique ginger soup. With all that ginger, garlic, onion, and other healthy ingredients, it will hopefully chase away any viruses that are headed your way.

1 tablespoon oil

⅔ cup ginger, peeled and minced

1 medium onion, peeled and chopped

1 teaspoon minced garlic

¼ teaspoon ground cardamom

¼ teaspoon ground cumin

3 cups chopped parsnips

3 cups chopped carrots

6 cups low-sodium vegetable or chicken broth

1 tablespoon honey

Salt and pepper

1½ cups heavy cream or milk

Yogurt or crème fraiche for serving, optional

Place oil in a large saucepan over medium heat. Add ginger, onion, garlic, cardamom, and cumin and cook, stirring frequently, for about 5 minutes or until quite soft and very aromatic. Do not allow the onion or garlic to take on any color.

Add parsnips and carrots, stirring to blend. Add broth along with the honey and season with salt and pepper. Raise heat and bring to a simmer. Lower heat to a gentle simmer, cover, and cook for about 30 minutes or until the vegetables are very tender.

Remove from heat and, using a hand-held immersion blender (or a blender or food processor fitted with the metal blade), process to a smooth puree.

Return soup to a clean pan and add the cream. Place over medium heat and bring to a bare simmer. Taste and, if necessary, season with salt and pepper.

Remove from heat and serve in shallow soup bowls with a dollop of plain yogurt or crème fraiche, if desired.

Salads

Roasted Chickpea Salad

SERVES 4

There are lots of recipes for pea and bean salads online, but we think this one is the best. It has a lovely combination of healthy flavors and colors.

    1 tablespoon olive oil

    4 cups cooked chickpeas, well drained

    1 teaspoon ground cumin

    1 teaspoon smoked paprika

    ½ teaspoon garam masala

    ½ teaspoon sea salt or to taste

    3 medium-sized carrots, peeled and finely diced

    1 hothouse cucumber (thin-skinned, such as English or
        Persian), trimmed and finely diced

    1 small red onion, peeled and finely diced

    ½ pound feta cheese, crumbled

    1 cup cilantro, mint, or basil leaves, plus more for garnish, if
        desired

    1 tablespoon fresh lemon juice

    1 tablespoon fresh orange juice

    1 teaspoon honey

    1 tablespoon extra virgin olive oil

    Salt and pepper

Heat the olive oil in a large frying pan over medium-high heat. Add the chickpeas and cook, stirring for about 2 minutes or just until the chickpeas are nicely coated in the oil. Add the cumin, paprika, garam masala, and salt and cook, stirring for about 10 minutes or until the chickpeas are nicely toasted and well coated in the spices. Remove from the heat and, using a slotted spoon, transfer to a double layer of paper towel to drain slightly.

Combine the carrot, cucumber, onion, feta, and herb leaves in a large mixing bowl. Add the lemon and orange juices, honey, and extra virgin olive oil. Season with salt and pepper.

Spoon an equal portion of the vegetable mixture into the center of each of four luncheon plates. Toss an equal amount of the warm chickpeas over the top of each and serve, garnished with additional herb leaves, if desired.

For a less fancy dish, you can toss the warm chickpeas into the vegetable mixture.

Kale-Quinoa Salad

SERVES 4 TO 6

You're likely to find this special Kale-Quinoa Salad divine with this citrus dressing. But don't stop there — these ingredients are so good for you, and the basic salad is so easy to make, that you'll want to try it two or three times, altering the accents until you love it. Throw in some dates, sliced almonds, or sesame or sunflower seeds. Or perhaps some chunks of ripe avocado, or bite-sized pieces from the orange that you zest for the dressing.

    1 cup quinoa (plain or multicolored)

    1 tablespoon olive oil

    1 medium onion, peeled and diced

    1 tablespoon minced garlic

    2 cups vegetable or chicken broth, or water

    Salt

    2 bunches kale

    1 cup toasted pumpkin seeds

    Pepper

    Citrus Dressing (recipe follows)

Place the quinoa in a fine-mesh sieve and rinse under cold running water until the water runs clear. Set aside to drain well.

Heat oil in a medium saucepan over medium heat. Add onion and garlic and cook, stirring occasionally, for about 5 minutes or until just beginning to color. Stir in the quinoa and then add the broth or water and season with salt. Raise the heat and bring to a boil. Cover, lower the heat, and cook for about 15 minutes or until the broth has been absorbed. Remove from heat and set aside to steam for about 5 minutes.

While the quinoa is cooking, prepare the kale. Pull off the tough stems from each leaf. Then cut the leaves into thin strips and place in a large salad bowl.

When the quinoa is ready, pour it over the kale and, using your hands (use thick rubber gloves to keep your hands from burning), toss the quinoa along with the pumpkin seeds into the kale. It is important that the quinoa be hot so that it wilts and tenderizes the kale. When just about totally combined, add just enough vinaigrette to season nicely and continue to toss and blend. Taste and season with salt and pepper.

Serve at room temperature.

Citrus Dressing

MAKES ABOUT 1 CUP

5 tablespoons rice wine vinegar

1 tablespoon fresh orange juice

1 tablespoon mirin (Japanese sweet rice wine)

½ tablespoon tamari

1 teaspoon ginger juice

Grated zest of 1 orange

2 tablespoons white miso paste (shiro miso)

6 tablespoons canola oil

Salt and pepper to taste

Combine the vinegar, orange juice, mirin, tamari, and ginger juice in a jar with a lid. Cover and shake to blend. Uncover, add the orange zest and miso, and, again, shake to blend. Open, add the canola oil, re-cover, and shake to emulsify. Taste and, if desired, season with salt and pepper.

Note: Although the Citrus Vinaigrette is delectable, you can use any vinaigrette or salad dressing you have on hand.

Snacks and Sides

Bonnie's Morning Veggies

SERVES 4–5

Bonnie has been relying on this delicious and nourishing snack for decades to ensure she gets enough vegetables every day.

Prep time: 15 minutes for 5 days of snacks

> ON THE WEEKEND, ADD THE FOLLOWING TO A LARGE MIXING BOWL:
>
> About 2 cups bite-size pieces of raw carrots
> About 2 cups sugar snap peas, cut into bite-size pieces
> About 2 cups bite-size pieces cut from peeled turnips
> About 2 cups chopped purple cabbage
> Any other raw veggie you like — radishes are one of her
>   favorites

Toss to combine the vegetables and divide the mix into 4 or 5 storage containers. Transfer to the refrigerator. When you are getting ready for work, spoon some into a lunch container, drizzle with a little extra virgin olive oil, and sprinkle with a tiny bit of salt.

Energy Bars

MAKES 12 BARS

These are the handiest, tastiest, healthiest snack bars imaginable. And you can adjust the berries and types of nut butter till you find the combination that your own family loves.

2 cups rolled oats

1 cup pumpkin seeds

1 cup sesame seeds

2 tablespoons chia seeds

½ cup brown sugar

½ cup almond butter

⅓ cup peanut butter

¼ cup honey

½ teaspoon ground cinnamon

½ cup dried cherries or cranberries

½ cup yellow raisins

Preheat the oven to 325°F.

Line a rimmed cookie sheet with parchment paper. Set aside.

Combine the oats with the pumpkin, sesame, and chia seeds on the cookie sheet. Place in the preheated oven and toast, stirring frequently, for about 12 minutes or until fragrant and lightly toasted.

While mixture is toasting, combine the brown sugar, almond butter, peanut butter, honey, and cinnamon in a small saucepan. Place over medium heat and, stirring frequently, bring to a simmer. Simmer for about 4 minutes or until the mixture is very smooth. Remove from heat.

When seeds are toasted, transfer to a large mixing bowl. Add cherries or cranberries and raisins and toss to blend.

Pour the warm butter mixture over the oat mixture and, working quickly, toss to blend completely. The mixture will set quickly so you must work with speed.

Scrape mixture into the baking pan with parchment paper. Using the palm of your hand, push mixture into a smooth, even layer.

Transfer to refrigerator and cool for about 3 hours or until firm enough to cut. Then use a serrated knife to cut into 12 bars of equal size.

Store, airtight, at room temperature.

Green Smoothie

MAKES ABOUT 12 OUNCES

There are so many green smoothies to choose from, but this one has a uniquely delicious combination of ginger and lemon.

> 2 stalks celery, trimmed and cut into chunks
> 1 small frozen banana, cut into chunks
> 1 Persian cucumber (or ½ an English cucumber), cut into
> chunks
> 1 cup chopped kale leaves
> 1 cup baby spinach leaves
> 1 teaspoon minced ginger or to taste
> Juice of ½ lemon
> About ½ cup unsweetened almond milk or any other milk of
> your choice

Combine celery, banana, cucumber, kale, spinach, and ginger in a blender jar. Process on high speed to blend thoroughly. Add lemon juice along with enough milk to make a smooth mix and again process on high until completely blended.

Serve immediately or store, covered and refrigerated, for no more than 12 hours. The mixture may separate slightly when stored, so when ready to serve, process in a blender until smooth.

Note: Try other fruits you have on hand — maybe that pear that is getting a bit ripe?

A Different Hummus

MAKES ABOUT 1½ CUPS

This is the dip that will make your family want to eat lots of raw veggies. And it takes only a few minutes to add this healthy, delicious recipe to your repertoire.

1 cup frozen petite peas, thawed and patted dry
¼ cup cilantro leaves
2 tablespoons tahini (sesame seed paste)
1 teaspoon minced garlic
½ teaspoon ground cumin
1½ tablespoons lemon juice
About 1 tablespoon extra virgin olive oil
Salt
Chile flakes

Combine peas, cilantro, tahini, garlic, and cumin in the bowl of a food processor fitted with the metal blade. Begin processing and, with the motor running, add the lemon juice and olive oil and process to a slightly chunky mixture. Season with salt and chile flakes and add just enough additional olive oil to thicken.

If the mixture seems too thick to use as a dip, thin with cool water one teaspoon at a time until you reach the consistency you want.

Serve immediately or scrape into a nonreactive container, cover, and refrigerate for up to 2 days.

Serve at room temperature with crisp pita chips or raw vegetables.

Mixed Cabbage Roast

SERVES 4 TO 6

Our ancestors would have considered this to be a comfort food — root vegetables with some exotic seasoning.

2½-pound cabbage, trimmed and cut into quarters or smaller

1½ pounds Brussels sprouts, trimmed and halved

⅓ cup olive oil

3 tablespoons lemon juice

3 tablespoons pure maple syrup

2 teaspoons lemon zest

Salt and pepper

Preheat the oven to 350°F.

Combine cabbage quarters and Brussels sprouts in a baking pan, preferably nonstick.

Combine olive oil, lemon juice, maple syrup, and lemon zest in a small bowl, beating to blend. When blended, pour mixture over the vegetables, taking care to cover evenly. Season with salt and pepper.

Transfer the vegetables to the preheated oven and roast, turning occasionally, for about 30 minutes or until just beginning to color.

Increase oven temperature to 400°F and continue to roast for another 15 minutes or until golden brown.

Stuffed Sweet Potatoes

SERVES 4

This recipe is a very clever combination of sweet potatoes and seasoned black beans. It could be an entrée for dinner or lunch, or a side dish with other meals. The sweet potatoes are so creamy after baking, and the bean combination is lovely with shredded cheese.

4 medium sweet potatoes, well scrubbed and dried

1 tablespoon plus 1 teaspoon olive oil

1 medium onion, peeled and finely diced

½ teaspoon minced garlic

1 cup cooked black beans, well drained

½ cup diced tomatoes, well drained

½ teaspoon ground cumin

½ teaspoon chili powder

Salt and pepper

Hot sauce to taste

Cilantro to taste

1 cup shredded Monterey Jack or sharp cheddar cheese

Heat oven to 375°F.

Prick potatoes in random spots with tines of a kitchen fork. Using 1 table-spoon of the oil, generously coat each one. Place on a cookie sheet lined with parchment paper or foil, put into the preheated oven, and bake for about 45 minutes or until very tender in the center when pierced with the end of a small sharp knife. Do not turn off the oven.

While the potatoes are cooking, make the filling.

Heat the remaining teaspoon of oil in a medium frying pan on medium heat. Add onion and garlic and cook, stirring frequently, for about 4 min-utes or just until softened. Add beans, tomatoes, cumin, and chili powder and continue to cook, stirring frequently, for about 10 minutes or just until the flavors have blended and most of the liquid has evaporated. Season with salt, pepper, and hot sauce. Remove from heat.

When the potatoes are cooked through, remove from the oven. Care-fully cut each one open by making a slash down the center without cutting through each end. Using your hand, push the potato open to make a slight hollow. Spoon an equal portion of the bean mixture into each hollow and then sprinkle an equal portion of the cheese over the beans.

Transfer potatoes to a baking sheet and place into the hot oven. Bake for about 10 minutes or until the cheese has melted.

Remove from oven, sprinkle with fresh cilantro, and serve immediately.

Also excellent as a side dish with something like the Beautiful Green Frit-tata found on page 203, or a green salad.

Main Courses

Julia's Easy and Portable Lunch

SERVES 1

Many people eat at work and don't have time or can't go out for lunch. This is one of Julia's most practical suggestions, as these are all items you can easily mix together at home in the morning or even the night before for a delicious lunch. This is designed as a single serving, but it's easy to scale up as desired. Dress the salad right before eating so that it doesn't get soggy.

Prep time: 5 minutes.

IN A LUNCH CONTAINER, PLACE YOUR SELECTIONS FROM THE FOLLOWING:

1–2 handfuls of leafy greens (spinach, kale, lettuce)

1 tomato, cut as desired

Watercress

1 carrot or beet, grated

¼–½ avocado, sliced or cubed

Protein choice: 2–3 ounces of canned tuna, leftover meat or fish (see Mix and Match Mains, page 228), or smoked salmon; 1–2 peeled and chopped boiled eggs; or 2–3 falafel balls

Cheese choice: 1–2 ounces of ricotta, Brie, or cheddar

3–5 olives

3–5 seeded crackers, and/or ¼ cup of leftover pasta or beans

Up to 10 nuts (cashews, almonds)

Add a splash of olive oil, and lemon juice or vinegar if you like. Mix well.

Voilà, you have lunch!

Moroccan-Spiced Black Bean Stew

SERVES 4 TO 6

This is no ordinary stew. It has such a range of nutrients, of textures, and of colors, and is even better on the second day.

2 tablespoons olive oil

1 large red onion, peeled and finely chopped

1 stalk celery, trimmed and finely chopped

1 teaspoon minced garlic

Chile flakes to taste

Salt

1 large sweet potato, peeled and cut into small cubes

1 small carrot, peeled and cut into small cubes

1 red bell pepper, cored, seeded, and cut into small cubes

1½ teaspoons ground coriander

1½ teaspoons ground cumin

1 teaspoon ground turmeric

¼ teaspoon ground cinnamon

5 cups low-sodium vegetable or chicken broth

One 28-ounce can chopped tomatoes with their juice

2 cups cooked black beans

About 1½ teaspoons soy sauce

Ground black pepper

2 tablespoons chopped cilantro, optional

Heat oil in a soup pot over medium heat. Add onion, celery, garlic, and chile flakes. Season with salt and cook, stirring frequently, for about 7 minutes or until the vegetables have begun to soften.

Add sweet potato, carrot, and bell pepper and stir to incorporate. Season with the coriander, cumin, turmeric, and cinnamon, stirring to blend. Add the broth, followed by the tomatoes and beans. Bring to a simmer. Taste and season with soy sauce and black pepper. Continue to simmer for about 20 minutes or until the stew is thick and the flavors have blended.

Serve hot, sprinkled with cilantro, if desired.

Note: This is particularly delicious served with soft flatbreads, such as naan or pita, for dipping into the rich sauce. The stew can also be served over rice or small noodles.

Peasant Lentil Stew

SERVES 4 TO 6

Feeling rushed for dinner, but wanting to cook something very nutritious? This basic recipe is for you. If you have dried lentils and basics like garlic on hand, then just grab some spinach or Swiss chard on the way home from work, and you'll have a wonderful supper.

2½ cups lentils (any color will work)

1 tablespoon olive oil

2 cloves garlic, peeled and minced

½ teaspoon chile flakes

2 stalks celery, trimmed and finely chopped

4 cups chopped spinach, kale, or Swiss chard

2 cups tomato sauce

1 teaspoon dried oregano

1 teaspoon dried basil

Salt and pepper

Place the lentils in a fine-mesh strainer and pick through to remove any small stones or debris. Rinse under cold running water until the water runs clear.

Transfer lentils to a large saucepan. Add 6 cups of cold water and place over high heat. Bring to a boil; then lower the heat and cook at a gentle simmer for 45 minutes.

While lentils are cooking, heat oil in a large frying pan over medium heat. Add garlic and chile flakes and fry, stirring frequently, for about 2 minutes or just until garlic begins to color slightly. Add celery and spinach (or other greens) and cook, stirring frequently, for about 10 minutes or until the vegetables have softened.

When the lentils have cooked for 45 minutes, scrape the vegetable mixture into them. Add the tomato sauce, oregano, and basil. Season with salt and pepper and continue to cook for an additional 15 minutes or until the flavors have blended and a rich, thick stew has formed.

Remove from the heat and serve.

Zucchini Tostadas

SERVES 4

Who doesn't love tostadas? But have you ever tried them with zucchinis? You will love having this delicious source of vegetables in your repertoire.

2 teaspoons olive, avocado, or canola oil

1 pound zucchini, trimmed and cut, crosswise, into slices

1 red bell pepper, trimmed, seeded, and diced

½ cup chopped sweet onion

2 teaspoons chili powder

½ teaspoon ground cumin

¼ teaspoon oregano

Salt and pepper

1 cup cooked black or pinto beans, well drained

4 corn or flour tortillas, warmed

½ cup shredded Monterey Jack cheese or cheddar cheese

Heat oil in a large frying pan over medium heat. Add zucchini, bell pepper, and onion. Season with chile powder, cumin, oregano, salt, and pepper, and cook, stirring occasionally, for about 7 minutes or until vegetables are still a bit crisp and the flavors have blended. Add the beans and cook for another minute or two or just until the beans are heated through.

Place an equal portion of the vegetable mixture on top of each tortilla. Sprinkle with the shredded cheese and serve.

Variations: The tostadas may be topped with shredded lettuce, chopped tomato, and/or your favorite salsa.

Chicken-Spinach Burgers

SERVES 4

Tired of hamburgers? Or even plain spinach burgers? Try this wonderful combination of greens and lemon for your next burger night.

> 1 pound ground skinless chicken breast or a mixture of breast
>   and thigh meat
> 1½ cups finely chopped fresh spinach leaves
> ¼ cup chopped flat leaf parsley
> ¼ cup minced scallion or sweet onion
> ½ teaspoon minced garlic
> ¼ teaspoon dried thyme
> 1 large egg white
> ¼ cup fresh breadcrumbs
> Salt and pepper
> About 1 tablespoon olive oil
> Lemon wedges for serving, optional

Place chicken in a medium mixing bowl. Add spinach, parsley, scallion, garlic, and thyme and stir to blend. Add egg white and breadcrumbs, season with salt and pepper, and, using your hands, mash the mixture together to blend thoroughly.

Form the mixture into four patties of equal size.

Heat oil in a large frying pan over medium heat. When hot, but not smoking, add patties.

Cook, turning occasionally, for about 12 minutes or until cooked through and a meat thermometer inserted into the center reads 160°F.

Remove from the pan and serve with a lemon wedge or on a bed of mixed greens or spinach, if desired.

Turkey Scallopini with Green Salad

SERVES 4

Another fresh take on how to present meat as your protein, but with lots of healthy greens in addition. This texture is extremely enticing if you haven't made turkey cutlets before.

Four 5-ounce turkey breast cutlets

2 large eggs

¼ cup milk

1½ cups breadcrumbs (plain or seasoned, depending upon your
    preference)

½ cup all-purpose flour

Salt and pepper

¼ cup olive oil plus more for dressing

4 loosely packed cups baby arugula (or other small salad green),
    well washed and dried

3 loosely packed cups baby spinach leaves

Juice of ½ lemon

Lemon quarters for serving

Place each turkey cutlet between 2 sheets of waxed or parchment paper. Working with one piece at a time and using a small, heavy frying pan or meat mallet, pound the meat out to about ⅛-inch thickness.

Combine eggs and milk in a shallow dish, whisking to blend well.

Combine breadcrumbs and flour in another shallow dish. Season with salt and pepper and stir to blend.

Working with one cutlet at a time, dip meat into the egg mixture, allowing excess to drip off. Then, dip it into the breadcrumb mixture. If you prefer a heavy coating, again dip into the egg and breadcrumb mixtures.

Heat ¼ cup of the olive oil in a large frying pan over medium-high heat. When very hot, but not smoking, add the cutlets, without crowding the pan. Fry, turning once, for about 5 minutes or until cooked through and crisp and golden brown on both sides. Transfer to a double layer of paper towel to drain.

Combine arugula and spinach in a mixing bowl and drizzle with about 2 tablespoons of olive oil and lemon juice. Season with salt and pepper and toss to coat.

Place a cutlet on each of 4 dinner plates. Mound an equal portion of the salad on top of the cutlets. If desired, serve with a lemon quarter for drizzling on the meat.

Stir-Fried Beef and Vegetables

SERVES 4

This is an excellent balance of vegetables, beef, nuts, and seeds, with Asian flavors. The Chinese five-spice powder makes this stir-fry extremely flavorful, and the red pepper on top is beautiful.

    3 tablespoons soy sauce

    3 tablespoons sherry wine

    1 tablespoon sesame oil

    1½ teaspoons Chinese 5-spice powder

    1 teaspoon minced garlic

    1 pound beef tenderloin or very lean beef stir-fry (e.g., flank
        steak), cut into thin strips

1 tablespoon peanut oil

2 cups broccoli florets

2 heads baby bok choy, trimmed and cut, crosswise, into pieces

1 red bell pepper, trimmed, seeded, and cut into strips

¼ cup chopped scallions

1 tablespoon sesame seeds

Ahead of time: Combine the soy sauce, sherry wine, sesame oil, 5-spice powder, and garlic in a bowl. Add the beef, and stir to coat evenly. Set aside to marinate for at least 15 minutes or up to 1 hour.

Heat peanut oil in a wok over high heat. When very hot, add the beef along with the marinade and the broccoli and stir-fry for about 4 minutes or just until the beef is barely cooked. Add bok choy and bell pepper and continue to stir-fry for 3 to 4 minutes or just until the beef is cooked through and the vegetables are still crisp-tender. Be careful not to overcook the beef.

Remove from heat and toss in scallions and sesame seeds.

Serve immediately with steamed rice, if desired.

Salmon with Green Lentils

SERVES 4

The Mediterranean diet suggests you eat fish at least twice a week, but it doesn't say the fish can't be fancy! Try this green lentil and vinegar/mustard dressing for your next salmon feast.

1½ cups dried green lentils

2 tablespoons red wine vinegar

1½ tablespoons grainy mustard

¼ cup extra virgin olive oil, plus 1 tablespoon

Salt and pepper

1 cup peeled, seeded, and diced tomato

3 tablespoons minced shallots

2 tablespoons minced flat leaf parsley

Four 5- to 6-ounce center-cut wild salmon filets

Place the lentils in a fine-mesh strainer and pick through to remove any small stones or debris. Rinse under cold running water until the water runs clear.

Transfer lentils to a large saucepan. Add 4 cups of cold water and place over high heat. Bring to a boil; then lower the heat and cook at a gentle simmer for 45 minutes or just until tender but still holding their shape.

While the lentils are cooking, combine the vinegar and mustard in a small mixing bowl. Whisk in ¼ cup olive oil and season with salt and pepper. Set aside until ready to use.

Preheat the oven to 400°F.

When tender, drain the lentils well and transfer to a medium mixing bowl. Add the tomato, shallots, and parsley, stirring to blend. Pour the dressing over the lentil mixture and gently toss to incorporate. Don't stir too vigorously as you want to keep the lentils whole. Set aside.

Season the salmon with salt and pepper.

Heat the remaining 1 tablespoon olive oil in a large ovenproof frying pan over medium-high heat. Add the salmon, skin side down, and sear for about 2 minutes or just until the skin is beginning to crisp.

Transfer to the preheated oven and roast for about 10 minutes or until the salmon is just barely cooked through. (You will need about 4 minutes per half inch of flesh for rare and about 6 minutes to cook completely.)

When ready to serve, spoon an equal portion of the lentils in the center of each of 4 dinner plates. Place a piece of salmon in the center of each plate and serve.

Pizza with Greens, Garlic, and Goat Cheese

SERVES 4

There has to be pizza in every diet, but no one said it had to be boring. Try this recipe that has multiple greens, goat cheese, and lovely balsamic flavors.

4 cups arugula leaves, well washed and dried

1 cup chopped radicchio

1 tablespoon chopped basil

1 tablespoon olive oil

1½ teaspoons Italian seasoning

Chile flakes to taste

One 12-inch prepared pizza base

2 tablespoons sliced or chopped black olives

1 tablespoon minced garlic

One 8-ounce goat cheese (chèvre) log, crumbled

Aged balsamic vinegar or balsamic glaze for drizzling

Preheat the oven to 450°F.

Place arugula, radicchio, and basil in a large mixing bowl. Add oil and seasoning and toss to coat. Season with chile flakes and toss again to distribute evenly.

Spread the seasoned greens over the pizza round. Sprinkle with olive slices and garlic and crumble the goat cheese over the top.

Transfer to a pizza stone or heavy-duty cookie sheet and place in preheated oven. Bake for about 10 minutes or until arugula has wilted and cheese melted. Remove from oven and drizzle with the balsamic.

Cut into wedges and serve piping hot.

Note: Possible substitutions for goat cheese are cream cheese or mascarpone. Or young children may prefer mozzarella.

Mix-and-Match Mains

And now it is time for you to use your own creativity to modify some recipes to suit your tastes and convenience. Here are some of our favorite variations on easy-and-fast roast chicken breast, fish recipes, and stir-fry recipes for meat or fish. Each serves two to four people and can be "dressed up" with your favorite hot sauce, served with greens or other vegetables, and/or accompanied by your best-loved rice or noodles. In other words, use your own ideas to make these easy variations useful for you!

Note: In all variations, mix the sauce ingredients together in a separate bowl before brushing onto the meat or fish.

Easy Baked Chicken Variations, Using 2 Boneless, Skinless Chicken Breasts

> 1 tablespoon olive oil
> 2 skinless, boneless chicken breast halves
> Salt and pepper
> Any one of the following wet or dry rubs

Preheat oven to 350°F.

Heat a tablespoon of olive oil in a medium frying pan over medium-high heat. Season the chicken with salt and pepper and carefully lay it into the hot oil. Sear, turning once, for about 4 minutes or just until the chicken is lightly browned and skin is sealed. This is to prevent the chicken from drying out while baking.

If using one of the wet rubs, such as Honey Mustard Chicken, using a pastry brush, lightly coat one side of the breast with half of wet rub before roasting.

If using a dry rub, such as the Sour Cream-Lime Chicken, using your hands, rub the mixture into both sides of the breasts before roasting.

For both methods, place the seared chicken in a small roasting pan. Transfer to the preheated oven and bake for 30 minutes. If using a wet rub, turn the breasts and, using the pastry brush, lightly coat with the remaining sauce. Continue to bake for another 10–15 minutes or until a meat thermometer inserted into the thickest part reads 165°F.

Serve with noodles or rice, with lots of vegetables on the side.

Note: You can replace chicken with pork loin, and it doesn't need to be seared. Cook it for 25 minutes per pound at 350°F.

Honey Mustard Chicken

    2 tablespoons olive oil

    2 teaspoons red wine vinegar

    2 teaspoons Dijon mustard

    1 teaspoon honey

    Pinch dried thyme and/or garlic powder

    Salt and pepper

Combine all of the ingredients in a small mixing bowl, stirring until very well blended. Use and roast as directed above for a wet rub.

or

Sour Cream-Lime Chicken

    2 teaspoons ground coriander

    1 teaspoon ground cumin

    Salt and pepper

    About 2 tablespoons sour cream or plain yogurt

    Juice of ½ lime

Combine the coriander and cumin and season with salt and pepper. Rub the mix into both sides of the chicken and bake as directed above for dry rub.

While the chicken is roasting, mix the sour cream or yogurt with the lime juice. When ready to serve, spoon the sour cream mixture onto the chicken breasts.

or

Chicken with Indian Seasoning

½ cup plain yogurt

1 teaspoon minced garlic

½ teaspoon grated ginger

½ teaspoon ground coriander

¼ teaspoon ground cumin

Juice of ½ lime

Lime wedges for serving, optional

Place the yogurt in a small mixing bowl. Add the garlic, ginger, coriander, and cumin, stirring to blend. Add the lime juice and stir to incorporate. Roast as directed above for wet rub. Serve with lime wedges, if desired.

or

Quick Creamy Chicken

4 tablespoons cream cheese, at room temperature

Pinch paprika

Place the cream cheese on a small plate and, using a rubber spatula, push to soften. Using a kitchen knife or sandwich spreader, carefully coat one side of each breast with softened cream cheese. Sprinkle with paprika and bake as directed for dry rub. Serve with a garnish of cilantro or on a bed of greens.

or

Pesto Chicken

3 cups basil leaves

3 cloves garlic, peeled and chopped

½ cup grated Parmesan cheese

3 tablespoons pine nuts

⅓ cup olive oil

¼ teaspoon salt

¼ teaspoon pepper

Combine the basil leaves with the garlic, Parmesan cheese, and pine nuts in the bowl of a food processor fitted with the metal blade. Process, using quick on and off turns, until finely chopped. With the motor running, add the olive oil in a slow steady stream, processing to an almost smooth puree. Season with salt and pepper and scrape into a clean container.

If not using immediately, place in a nonreactive container, smooth the top, and cover with a thin coat of olive oil. (This will keep the sauce from oxidizing.) Store, covered and refrigerated, for up to 1 week. Sauce can also be frozen for up to 3 months.

Pesto can either be spread on the chicken breasts as for a wet rub or it can be used as a side sauce with the roasted breasts. It is also a terrific sauce for pasta or grains.

If basil is not available, you can substitute kale or a mix of other strongly flavored greens.

Seafood Variations, Using About 12 Ounces Fish Filets, Scallops, or Shrimp

These variations are useful as marinades, so if you can, prepare the sauce ahead of time and allow the seafood to marinate in it for about 30–60 minutes to enhance the flavor.

Note: If you're using scallops or shrimp, they cook very quickly — usually in just a few minutes. You'll know they're done when the scallops are wholly opaque and the shrimp are pink.

Skillet-Poached Salmon with Indian Spices

1 teaspoon minced garlic

½ teaspoon garam masala

½ teaspoon ground coriander

½ teaspoon ground cumin

3 tablespoons olive oil

Salt and pepper

Two 6-ounce skinless salmon filets

Lemon or lime wedges for serving, optional

Combine the garlic, garam masala, coriander, and cumin in a small mixing bowl. Add the olive oil and season with salt and pepper. Stir to blend well.

Using your hands, coat both sides of the salmon with the spice mix.

Place the seasoned salmon in a nonstick frying pan over low heat. Cook for 8 minutes, turning once, or until the salmon is just barely cooked through. You can add a tablespoon of water to the pan if it gets too dry.

Serve immediately with lemon or lime wedges, if desired.

Skillet Halibut with Thai Seasoning

    2 teaspoons olive oil

    ½ medium onion, peeled and diced

    2 teaspoons curry powder

    2 cups low-sodium chicken broth

    3½ ounces unsweetened coconut milk

    Salt and pepper

    Two 6-ounce halibut filets

Place the oil in a large frying pan over medium heat. Add the onion and cook, stirring frequently, for about 4 minutes or until the onion begins to soften. Stir in the curry powder and continue to cook, stirring, for about 4 more minutes. Add the chicken broth and coconut milk, season with salt and pepper, and bring to a simmer. Simmer for 5 minutes or until fragrant and slightly thick.

Add the halibut and spoon the sauce over it. Cover and cook for about 7 minutes or until the fish flakes easily when pierced with a kitchen fork.

Remove from the heat and serve with the sauce spooned over the top.

Oven-Roasted Salmon with Yogurt Sauce

    Two 6-ounce skin-on salmon filets

    Salt and pepper

    ½ cup plain yogurt

    1 tablespoon plus 2 teaspoons olive oil plus more for the pan

    1 tablespoon orange juice (squeezed from the orange you use
        for zesting)

    1 tablespoon minced flat leaf parsley

    1 tablespoon minced capers

    ½ teaspoon orange zest

Preheat the oven to 400°F.

Lightly coat a small roasting pan with 2 teaspoons of the olive oil. Set aside.

Season the salmon with salt and pepper. Place in the prepared roasting pan, skin side down, and transfer to the preheated oven. Roast for 15 minutes or until just cooked through.

While the salmon is roasting, prepare the sauce.

Place the yogurt in a small mixing bowl. Add the remaining 1 tablespoon olive oil along with the orange juice, parsley, capers, and orange zest. Season with salt and pepper and whisk to combine.

Remove the salmon from the oven, place on a serving platter, and drizzle with yogurt sauce. Serve immediately.

Stir-Fry Variations for 1 Pound Meat, Chicken, or Shrimp

In addition to the Stir-Fried Beef and Vegetables recipe on page 224, there are many sauces that work well for Asian meat and fish stir-fries. The variations below are designed for one pound of beef (thinly sliced flank steak, round steak, or sirloin), chicken (thinly sliced chicken breast), or shrimp.

Spicy Stir-Fry with Peanuts

    2 tablespoons soy sauce
    2 teaspoons fish sauce
    1 pound beef, chicken, or shrimp as described above
    1 tablespoon chile garlic sauce
    1 tablespoon lime juice
    1 tablespoon light brown sugar
    1½ teaspoons peanut oil
    ½ cup chopped unsalted peanuts
    ⅓ cup chopped cilantro

Combine 1 tablespoon soy sauce and 1 teaspoon fish sauce in a small bowl.

Place the protein in a medium shallow bowl and drizzle the sauce over the top, tossing to lightly coat. Set aside to marinate for 30 minutes.

Combine the remaining 1 tablespoon soy sauce and 1 teaspoon fish sauce with the chile garlic sauce, lime juice, and sugar, stirring to blend well. Set aside.

Place the peanut oil in a wok or large frying pan over medium-high heat. When very hot, but not smoking, add the protein. Stir-fry for 2 minutes. Add the reserved sauce and stir-fry for an additional 2 minutes.

Remove from the heat and serve as is or with steamed rice or rice noodles, garnished with the peanuts and cilantro.

Note: This recipe is also good with greens, such as chopped asparagus, peas, or spinach, added to the protein during the stir-fry.

Stir-Fried Beef and Broccoli

> 6 tablespoons soy sauce
>
> 3 tablespoons light brown sugar
>
> 2 tablespoons sesame oil
>
> 2 teaspoons minced garlic
>
> 1 teaspoon minced ginger
>
> 1½ tablespoons cornstarch
>
> 1 tablespoon olive oil
>
> 6 cups broccoli florets
>
> 1 pound beef (thinly sliced flank steak, round steak, or sirloin),
>   or other desired protein

Combine the soy sauce, sugar, sesame oil, garlic, and ginger in a medium mixing bowl. Add ½ cup hot water and stir to blend. Stirring constantly, add the cornstarch, and continue to stir until it is completely dissolved. Set aside.

Heat the olive oil in a wok or large frying pan over medium-high heat. Add 2 tablespoons hot water along with the broccoli. Cover and allow the broccoli to steam for about 3 minutes or just until beginning to soften.

Uncover, add the protein along with the reserved sauce, and stir-fry for about 3 minutes or just until the protein is cooked through. You do not want to overcook or the broccoli will be soggy and the protein tough.

Serve as is or over steamed rice.

Desserts

Chocolate Beet Cake

MAKES ONE 8-INCH CAKE

This dessert is rich in flavor and nutrients, and the beets give it a surprising texture — no one will even know they're in there.

½ pound cooked beets

1 cup all-purpose flour

3 tablespoons 100% cacao cocoa powder

1¼ teaspoons baking powder

7 ounces bittersweet (at least 60% cacao) chocolate, chopped
        into small pieces

2 teaspoons pure vanilla extract

3.5 ounces butter, at room temperature, cubed

5 large eggs, at room temperature, separated

1 cup brown sugar

Preheat the oven to 350°F.

Lightly butter and flour an 8-inch springform or cake pan.

Cut beets into pieces, place them in a blender, and purée until smooth; or, if you like a bit more texture in your cake, just chop the beets finely with a food processor. Set aside.

Combine flour, cocoa powder, and baking powder and sift into a medium mixing bowl. Set aside.

Place chocolate in top half of a double boiler set over simmering water. Heat, stirring occasionally, for about 4 minutes or until it is almost melted. Add ¼ cup hot water along with the vanilla, remove pan from heat, and stir to blend completely. Add the butter pieces and, without stirring, let them begin to melt into the chocolate.

Remove pan with melted chocolate from the double boiler and, using a wooden spoon, beat to completely blend in the melting butter. Continue stirring occasionally to allow mixture to cool slightly.

While mixture cools slightly, beat the egg whites in a standing electric mixer (or with a hand-held electric mixer) until soft peaks form. Sprinkle in the sugar and continue to beat until stiff peaks form and sugar is fully incorporated into the whites.

Gently fold the reserved flour mixture into the beaten egg whites.

When chocolate has cooled slightly, using a whisk, beat in egg yolks. Then add the reserved beets by gently folding them into the batter with a spatula. Finally, add chocolate mixture by folding into flour and beet mixture.

Scrape batter into prepared pan and place in the preheated oven. Bake for 5 minutes. Then reduce the heat to 325°F and continue to bake for about 30 minutes or until sides of the cake seem firm but center remains shaky. Do not overbake or the cake will be dry. It will continue to firm as it cools.

Remove from oven and let it cool completely on a wire rack before removing from cake pan and serving.

Nutty Black Bean Brownies

MAKES ABOUT 1 DOZEN

Who would have thought you could make brownies with beans? Even better, the kids won't even know they're in there! And on top of that, it's full of antioxidant-rich dark chocolate. This is also a great choice for vegans.

1½ cups cooked black beans, very well drained

½ cup quick-cooking regular oats

⅓ cup light brown sugar

¼ cup 100% cacao cocoa powder

¼ cup coconut oil

1 teaspoon pure vanilla extract

1 teaspoon instant espresso powder

½ teaspoon baking powder

½ teaspoon baking soda

1 cup dark chocolate (at least 60% cacao) chips

1 cup chopped walnuts, almonds, peanuts, or pecans

Preheat oven to 350°F.

Lightly butter and flour an 8-inch by 8-inch baking pan. Set aside.

Combine beans with oats, sugar, and cocoa powder in the bowl of a food processor fitted with the metal blade. Add oil, vanilla, espresso powder, baking powder, and baking soda and process until very, very smooth. The texture will influence the final taste so it is important to make sure the mixture is lump-free and liquidy smooth.

Pour mixture into a mixing bowl and stir in the chocolate chips and nuts.

Scrape mixture into the prepared pan. Transfer to preheated oven and bake for about 25 minutes or until firm.

Remove from oven and place on a wire rack to cool before cutting into squares and serving.

10

FOODS TO AVOID FOR A BETTER BRAIN

NOW THAT YOU KNOW the best way to eat, you also need to know why it's so difficult for most consumers to actually make informed choices. Nutritionists tell us that eggs are bad for us — but then they're not. Or are they? Fat-free foods suddenly blossom on supermarket shelves, with few people realizing that the fat was swapped with sugar, and that's why they were unwittingly gaining weight.

All of this food information is still targeted toward your physical health — but what about your mental health? Let's take a look at what you want to avoid, and what guidelines you might want to consult.

Dietary Guidelines: Does Your Government Really Care What You Eat?

Governments all over the world produce their own dietary guidelines. These are important even if the general population is not terribly well informed about their own country's guidelines, because those guidelines influence how every institution purchases and prepares the food they provide. This means that the food provided in schools, hospitals, prisons, nursing homes, and so on is influenced by these guidelines, especially if that institution receives any government funding.

In the United States, an advisory committee is established every five years to review all the scientific evidence, and then a new set of dietary guidelines is produced. The current American guidelines, as published on the health.gov website, states that a healthy eating pattern *includes*:

- A variety of vegetables from all of the subgroups — dark green, red and orange, legumes (beans and peas), starchy, and other
- Fruits, especially whole fruits
- Grains, at least half of which are whole grains
- Fat-free or low-fat dairy, including milk, yogurt, cheese, and/or fortified soy beverages
- A variety of protein foods, including seafood, lean meats and poultry, eggs, legumes (beans and peas), and nuts, seeds, and soy products
- Oils

A healthy eating pattern *limits*:

- Saturated fats and trans fats, added sugars, and sodium

As you can see, Americans are currently being told to eat a diet that actually resembles the Mediterranean diet (although they don't use that label). The biggest difference is that the actual Mediterranean diet says to consume olive oil, and the American guidelines just say oils.

Many of us still think about this guideline in terms of the food pyramid or servings per day, both of which are reasonable approaches still utilized in many countries. The problem, however, is that few people know what a serving is! Is it a cup? A half cup? During a continuing medical education lecture to family doctors, Bonnie asked the audience to define a serving. They didn't know. This knowledge gap was a wake-up call for these doctors, as they realized that if they didn't know, how could they counsel their patients?

In a move that seems much more practical than expecting people to know what a serving size is, a few countries have dropped the serving/ day recommendations in their guidelines and instead recommend food according to plate size. As we've mentioned, half of your plate should be filled with fruits and vegetables, and the other half with a mix of protein, fats, and complex carbohydrates. Of course, then the question for people focused on the obesity epidemic is: Well, how big is your plate?! Did you know that the American plate size has increased from eight and a half inches (which holds 800 calories) in the 1960s to twelve inches (which can hold 1,900 calories) in the twenty-first century? Lesson is — use a smaller plate!

According to the Food and Agriculture Organization of the United Nations, over one hundred countries have established dietary guidelines (you can look for your country here: http://www.fao.org/nutrition/ education/food-dietary-guidelines/home/en/). All appear to emphasize *variety,* adequate *water,* and lots of *fruits and vegetables.* The US image on ChooseMyPlate.Gov shows vegetables as the largest component. Canada's plate puts vegetables and fruit together, taking up 50 percent of the plate — and leaves out *all* dairy, which caused an uproar in the dairy industry! The Eatwell Guide from the United Kingdom, the German Nutrition Circle, and the Argentina graphic employ similar imagery. But in addition to the older pyramid style and the newer plate-based imagery, many countries like New Zealand and Brazil still depend on written, descriptive guidelines.

Dietary guidelines can become politicized and controversial. For instance, there are many who feel that the American emphasis on low-fat content and lean meat is highly misplaced. This feeling stems from food manufacturers replacing fat with sugar, which quickly led to weight gain. And if you think about what your grandparents or great-grandparents ate, full fat was a normal part of their diet. Skim milk was unheard of. Low-fat cheese and yogurt hadn't been invented. Butter was on practically every table. Yet those generations didn't come close to having the obesity levels we see in countries around the globe right now (or the high rate of mental health issues).

Many authors have written diet books on this topic, but the research hasn't shown that eating a low-fat diet leads to better health. Others write about reducing or cutting meat out of their diets completely. While it is important to focus on the environmental damage and carbon emissions that come from some agricultural practices, we know how important it may be to still eat *some* meat for better mental health, especially if the animals are grass-fed rather than corn-fed (the latter being the norm in the United States). If you can't eat meat for health reasons or if doing so is contrary to your belief system (which is totally fine, of course), you need to replace protein and get your vitamin B12 and iron from other sources — which will require supplementation for some. (Refer to chapter 11 for more.) We think it's possible to find a balance between trying to save our planet and optimizing our health.

What Not to Eat!

It's not just the *presence* of healthy food but also the *absence* of unhealthy food that contributes to a good outcome. Aside from individual sensitivities and preferences, what *not* to eat for optimal brain health goes back to eating real food first. Don't eat processed, packaged items that are labeled as food but are mostly a chemical soup in a can or a bag or a box. Eat true food instead.

Hopefully, the following information will help you make better-informed choices about real food.

A Spoonful of Sugar . . .

According to the US Department of Health and Human Services, "Two hundred years ago, the average American ate only two pounds of sugar a year. In 1970, we ate 123 pounds of sugar per year. Today, the average American consumes almost 152 pounds of sugar in one year. This is equal to three pounds (or six cups) of sugar consumed in one week. Nutritionists suggest that Americans should get only 10 percent of their calories from sugar. This equals 13.3 teaspoons of sugar per day (based on 2,000 calories per day). The current average is 42.5 teaspoons of sugar per day!"

You can see why sugar has been demonized for quite a few decades — we're simply eating too much of it. But don't forget that our brains need glucose to function, so we need to get some type of sugars from our diet. Our ancestors got most of their sugar from real foods, like fruit, which naturally limited the amount they could consume. Now that we have endless tempting bags and boxes of sugary treats available 24/7 that can provide us with the sugar of *thirty* oranges in one hit, well, you can do the math! Added to the mix is that many foods you wouldn't expect (like peanut butter) are "fortified" with high fructose corn syrup, exponentially increasing the amount of sugar our bodies receive.

Can we attribute hyperactivity to sugar consumption? This topic is highly controversial, but the data tell us that no, not in the short term (a few hours). Even kids who are said to be sugar-reactive are no more likely to respond to sugar challenges under controlled conditions. In fact, some studies show that in the short term, sugar can improve cognitive function! So when kids are hyper at a party, it might be because they are hanging out with their friends and having lots of fun, and the consumption of cakes and candies brings along a host of artificial additives that we know cause behavior problems in some children (see chapter 4). Studies show, however, that parents who *think* their child has consumed sugar will rate them as more hyperactive than if they aren't told their child has consumed sugar. That's the power of having a strong expectation.

Are we saying it's okay to eat lots of highly refined sugar? Of course not! *Especially not long term.* Back in the 1980s, researchers looking at the role that sugar and other refined foods lacking nutrients played in antisocial behaviors in children and adolescents saw that over a three-month period, there was almost a 45 percent reduction in disciplinary actions in the kids who had reduced their sugar compared with those who didn't.[1] Based on this research, reducing chronic sugar consumption would hopefully make a difference across a range of challenging behaviors.

And, of course, some candy is okay once in a while. When you eat a mainly healthy diet, enjoy your occasional treats, and the pleasure it will bring to your kids.

Drinks to Avoid

Coke Zero is a great name for that drink — it has *zero* nutrients! That in itself should be a good reason to reduce or even eliminate your soda consumption, along with energy drinks, sport drinks, and other sugary drinks. A twenty-ounce bottle of soda contains the equivalent of sixteen sugar cubes. You're not about to dissolve that much sugar into a glass of water and drink it!

Plain water should be your primary source of fluid. Try flavoring with a few slices of lime or orange, and you won't miss soda at all. For someone transitioning from sugared soda to water, a good interim drink is carbonated water or seltzer, either adding a few slices of fruit, buying sugar-free bottled or canned seltzer, or making your own with a SodaStream device. The intermediary step helps you wean off sugar while still enjoying a bubbly drink.

Be careful, too, about making your smoothies too sweet, a common mistake. Or putting a lot of sugar in your tea or coffee. If you stick to green and herbal teas, you won't want sugar at all!

Is Coffee Good for You?

Coffee is one of the most studied compounds on earth — enter the word "coffee" into a search of the medical-literature website Medline and over

15,000 studies will pop up. And it's probably safe to say that every single investigator was looking in part for potential problems linked to coffee consumption. Yet in all these years of scientific research, no one has ever found one to two cups of daily coffee to be significantly harmful for our health.

The exception, of course, is if someone has a genetic vulnerability that makes it hard for them to metabolize coffee, as well as the fact that caffeine makes some people feel anxious or have trouble sleeping. If anxiety or insomnia is a challenge for you, then you might want to stop caffeine for a few months to see if that helps. Also, some people feel that their heart is sensitive to caffeine, and its rhythm changes. Others find coffee aggravates gastrointestinal problems. Again, leave coffee off the menu (or try decaf) and observe if it makes a difference.

In general, our addiction to a morning cup of coffee doesn't seem to be harmful to most people's mental (or physical) health. And let's acknowledge that it even contains some nutrients! Not a lot, but a single cup of coffee does usually provide tiny amounts of four vitamins and three minerals.

Why Ultra-Processed Food Is So Bad for You

All food that has been placed in bottles, cans, boxes, or bags is "processed" in some way to prevent spoilage. But there is an enormous difference between a can of San Marzano tomatoes that you might use in your home-made spaghetti sauce and a can of ravioli sweetened with high fructose corn syrup.

There are many reasons why a diet high in processed food is bad for your body. Processed food tends to be high in sugars and unhealthy fats like trans fats, which often lead to weight gain and all the problems that can arise as a result. Also, they usually contain excessive amounts of sodium. According to the American Heart Association, "more than 70 percent of the sodium Americans eat comes from packaged, prepared, and restaurant foods — not the salt shaker." This can lead to high blood pressure, heart disease, and strokes. These items are also low in fiber, probably accounting for a significant amount of constipation.

Processed food also affects the health of your brain. As we mentioned in chapter 2, recent results from the SUN study found a relationship between shorter telomere length and quantity of ultra-processed food consumed by 886 older adults. The common denominator is, not surprisingly, that packaged/ultra-processed/prepared products are nutrient-poor foods, and whole/natural foods are more nutritious.

Absence of Nutrients

If you are eating a lot of processed food, then you are not getting enough of the minerals, vitamins, omega-3 fatty acids, and phytonutrients that are good for you, despite the nutrient fortification you might see on a label. Fortification consists of the addition of only a few nutrients and only at the doses required to prevent a frank nutritional deficiency disease such as rickets or scurvy. Replacing good nutrients with processed food that might temporarily fill your stomach does not adequately feed your brain. So without a doubt, the major harm that occurs from depending on ultra-processed products to fill your stomach is that you are choosing NOT to consume the minerals and vitamins and essential fatty acids that your brain needs every minute of every day.

Chemicals in Our Food and the Precautionary Principle

Many processed foods contain a lot of chemicals, including artificial colors and preservatives, some of which may be harming your brain. Of these tens of thousands of chemicals in our food supply, some 5,000 are in a category sometimes referred to as PFAS (per- and poly-fluoroalkyl substances) — toxic fluorinated or "forever chemicals" — because they do not get metabolized or broken down or washed away. According to a report released by the Environmental Working Group in January 2020, their "scientists now believe PFAS is likely detectable in all major water supplies in the U.S., almost certainly in all that use surface water. EWG's tests also found chemicals from the PFAS family that are not commonly tested for in drinking water."

Few consumers could know which chemicals are present, or we are fooled by them being labeled "natural flavors," "all-natural," or "antioxidant." (Never mind that snake venom and poison ivy are also "all-natural"!)

In general, the public needs to understand that companies are free to add many chemicals that have not been proven to be safe. That's right! This is the opposite of what a cautious approach would be — proving a chemical is safe *before* adding it to our food supply. But that approach, called the Precautionary Principle, is *not* followed in many Western governments, including in the United States.

What's desperately needed is funding for thousands and thousands of studies rigorously looking into the chemicals that are already in our food supply. Those studies should go beyond determining whether the chemicals cause cancer or other diseases. Research investigating the association between low-level pesticide exposure and psychiatric disorders highlights the complexity of determining risk but also suggests there may be some people who are more vulnerable to pesticide exposure than others.[2]

Yet these studies are not likely to happen. Why? Because it's very difficult to get funding for such work. The food industry is not going to pay for it, and neither are governments. That's not to say that governments don't try to monitor safety and/or do some in-house testing — they do! But it seems to be a drop in the bucket compared to what's needed. Add to that the problem of the cocktail effect: While one chemical might be okay to consume, what about consuming different combinations? Could combinations and interactions be a problem? If so, then studying one chemical at a time isn't going to tell us much about the overall health effects.[3]

This is why it's so difficult to know if there are any direct harmful effects of food chemicals on our brains. All that we can say is that improving your overall nutrition buffers the effects of exposure to harmful chemicals (as we explained in chapter 2), and that improving your nutrition protects you from many environmental harms as well.

A great initiative is the Dirty Dozen and Clean Fifteen list published each year by the Environmental Working Group (ewg.org). It helps consumers know which fruits and vegetables are likely to have a high pesticide content. This can then help direct which ones are better to buy as organic. The list changes from year to year but it is worth checking out. For example, strawberries often feature on the Dirty Dozen list as they have the highest level of residue and can contain dozens (!) of different types of pesticides. On the other hand, avocadoes are often on the Clean Fifteen list as they typically have a low level of pesticide residue.

Shortcuts/Easy Swaps

Many parents know that when their kids come home ravenous from school or an activity, they'll grab whatever's convenient. If you regularly offer raw veggies and hummus, or cut-up apples and oranges, they'll forget about potato chips or cookies. And you will feel reassured that you are giving your children the maximum nutrients possible when you provide raw veggies in addition to cooked.

But we all have cravings from time to time for something crunchy, or salty, or sweet. This list will give you better choices on the right for the processed food on the left.

Avoid This	Try This Instead
Baked goods	Trail mix, dried fruit
Chewy candy	Blueberries, dried raisins, dried apples
Chips, potato or corn	Air-popped popcorn, nuts, whole grain crackers with cheese
Dips, store-bought	Homemade Hummus (see recipe page 215)
French fries	Baked sweet-potato "fries"
Fried food	Food cooked in an air fryer or convection oven
Ice cream	Greek yogurt with fruit

Is Your Child a Picky Eater?
Try the Thank You Bite

The association between mood, anxiety, and diet has been shown in children as young as ten, as you know. The message is clear: we all need to help parents learn to feed their children a healthier diet.

This can be a problem for those children who have a strong aversion to some tastes and textures. No one knows this better than the parents of children on the autism spectrum, but many other children are picky eaters, too. Some cases can be really extreme. One child we know would only eat egg salad sandwiches made with Hellman's mayonnaise, and no other food, for years! (Another brand of mayonnaise led to screaming tantrums.) Some kids will only eat chicken fingers, or beige food. What to do?

First, keep trying to introduce different foods to your child. Don't give up when a food is initially rejected! We all know the feeling—maybe you balked at your first taste of cilantro or Brussels sprouts or parsnips. But after trying these foods many times, perhaps prepared with different cooking methods, sometimes you get used to or even start to love some of them. Many dietitians recommend at least ten attempts to help your child get used to a food.

The question for parents of picky eaters is how in the world to do that, especially if the child tends to spit it out with lots of drama and puking noises! (We're sure some of you know exactly what that's like.)

We suggest you try this tip from a physician who went to one of Bonnie's discussion groups many years ago; we'd love to credit her for this novel idea but Bonnie never caught her name. This technique is called the Thank You Bite. Let's say there are four veggies your child totally rejects. Every few days, put a small amount of one of them on your child's plate, and a small bowl next to the dinner plate. Explain that they are now expected to put one bite of the veggie into their mouth, chew it up, *but not swallow it*. He has to spit it into the bowl quietly and say, "Thank you."

How does this work? Over time, the children will hopefully get used to the taste of at least one of those veggies, just by chewing it. The Thank You bowl eliminates all the drama of the situation. Try to be very matter-of-fact in your presentation, and accept the possibility that success will take a long time. The stress reduction for all at the dinner table makes this definitely worth a shot.

Creating a Plan for Success

Change isn't easy, which is why scientists and researchers have spent decades investigating why people don't succeed in making changes they know will be good for their health. Professors James Prochaska and Carlo DiClemente and colleagues developed the transtheoretical model in the 1970s, originally developed to help understand why people couldn't/wouldn't stop addictive behaviors like drinking alcohol or smoking cigarettes. The Transtheoretical Model of Behavior Change has now been applied to dozens of health behaviors, including why people don't stop eating certain foods even when they know they're bad for them. These researchers identified that changing behaviors requires motivation and readiness, which occur in five steps:

Step 1: Pre-contemplation (not ready)

Step 2: Contemplation (getting ready)

Step 3: Preparation (ready)

Step 4: Action

Step 5: Maintenance

So how do we get ourselves launched successfully across these steps? We have a few tips to help you on this journey:

1. Start with tangible goals. Be specific about what you plan to do. Maybe start by changing what you eat for breakfast, or cooking two meals a week instead of getting takeout or ultra-processed foods. Perhaps you drink sugary sodas every day and you want to quit: consider tapering over several weeks. You can do so by drinking a soda only on Saturdays and Sundays; then the next week cutting that amount in half. Make sure whatever goal you choose is realistic and easily doable.

2. Consider *when* you are going to start. Make sure you don't set goals you simply can't achieve due to timing. If you know you're going to have house guests, a huge and stressful project at work, or a vacation coming up, this won't be the time to start shopping and cooking more than you usually do.

3. Many psychologists focus on making sure you are clear about your WHY. How does improving your diet help you achieve specific health goals? Does changing your diet align with making sure you are alive to see your grandchildren grow up?

4. Make sure you have support from others along the way. Sharing your plans and goals with trusted friends and family can help keep you committed and accountable to your intended changes. Having someone commit to making their own changes at the same time is also a good way to stay on track — you can support each other.

5. Be prepared for setbacks and how you'll deal with them. Know they will happen — you're only human! If you have a trigger food that you know you can't stop eating once you start (like potato chips or chocolate bars, or even certain cheeses that are nutritious in small quantities), try not to buy it very often. Don't beat yourself up because you ate a fast food meal — it's just a slip and not a reason to quit.

Another barrier that's really important to acknowledge is that when someone is depressed or struggling with other mental health challenges like addictions, getting the energy and motivation to make any changes in how and what they eat may seem insurmountable. If this is you, you might find that using nutrient supplements first, as you'll see in the next chapter, may get you to a good place mentally so that you're able to start considering changes to your diet.

The Takeaway

1. Government dietary guidelines are meant to help consumers figure out the healthiest way to eat, and they often change over time. Bottom line: the Mediterranean or whole foods diet *won't* change, so stick to the basics for optimal brain health.

2. Your brain requires some sugar for optimal functioning, but it's nowhere near the amount the average consumer eats. It's always best to get sugar from natural sources, like fruit.

3. Eating a diet high in processed foods means you are swapping out healthy real food for food that might be filling, but is low in the nutrients your brain needs. You are wasting your brain's potential as well as your money!

4. There are thousands of chemicals in highly processed food, and we just don't know how they affect our brain health, especially when combinations of them haven't been tested.

5. Changing your diet starts with the first step. Choose a goal and stick to it. Once mastered, move on to a new goal.

11

SUPPLEMENTS:
WHAT YOU NEED TO KNOW

IT'S ALWAYS BEST TO get your essential nutrients from whole foods, as you know already. But if you're doing your best to eat an excellent diet and are still having issues with your mental health or difficulty coping with stress, it might be time to consider adding a supplement.

We've both seen an interesting sequence for many people in this state of mind: they take nutrient supplements, feel better, realize that improving their nutrition is important for their mental health, and then work even harder to improve their diet.

When are supplements truly needed? They're most needed during times of intense stress, post-trauma, during pregnancy and postpartum, when you are struggling with serious mental health issues, and/or if you have a strong family history of mental health problems. This chapter will provide you with information on the multinutrient products that have been studied, including dose, nutrient/drug interactions, and where to buy them. We will also introduce you to the legislation that makes it hard for manufacturers to tell you about the health benefits on their labels, even when there is scientific proof of efficacy.

Before You Start: Testing Your Nutrient Levels

The question that is often on people's minds is whether they need to get their nutrients tested before they take supplements.

Others wonder whether it is worth trying supplementation if blood tests show that one or several of their nutrient levels are normal. And yet others might wonder if they should only take specific nutrients based on the ones identified as deficient on the tests. Will you still benefit from nutrients added to your already healthy diet?

The answer is quite simple — these blood tests are not necessary for deciding on treatment, nor are they generally helpful. Let's explain. When we look at whether pre-treatment information tells us if a person is going to respond to a treatment, we call that variable a *predictor*. Predictors can be useful to help decide which patients might be very likely to do well (or not). An example would be the VITACOG study we told you about in chapter 6. It was only the study participants with elevated levels of homocysteine (an amino acid) whose cognitive decline and brain atrophy slowed down when given the high doses of B vitamins. The predictor was their homocysteine levels at the onset of the study.

Julia's ADHD Studies

Julia's lab looked at whether blood levels of nutrients are *predictive* of how people would respond to broad-spectrum multinutrient supplements. Her studies treat *everyone,* regardless of their blood test results, and then assess whether nutrient levels predicted whose symptoms improved.

In two studies, pre-treatment blood levels of vitamin B12, vitamin D, zinc, copper, folate, ferritin, potassium, sodium, calcium, and homocysteine were checked. These are commonly part of regular blood tests for nutrient levels. She looked at two data sets — an adult study and a child study, both comparing broad-spectrum multinutrients with a placebo to treat ADHD symptoms. (Both these ADHD studies were described in chapter 5 where we told you that about half of the participants showed substantial benefit from the nutrient treatment.)

They looked for deficiencies identified *before* treatment, and they found that the vast majority of the nutrient levels fell in the normal range across both studies.[1]

Overall, nutrient levels before treatment did *not* reliably predict who would do well and who wouldn't. Pre-treatment nutrient levels also didn't show associations with any of the ADHD symptoms.

So the all-important question was asked: If your nutrient levels were "normal" when you started the study, did you benefit from taking the supplements? And the answer was yes! About 40 percent of those with "normal" nutrient levels benefited greatly when given broad-spectrum multinutrients.

Here is the most startling finding: family doctors usually decide whether to recommend supplements based on the results they see in your blood work. If a deficiency had been used as an inclusion criterion for this study, 72 *percent* of the group would never have gotten into the study in the first place — because their blood samples showed normal nutrient levels! This actually shouldn't be that surprising because the body works hard through homeostatic mechanisms to keep many (but not all) nutrient levels within a narrow range.

So almost three-quarters of the participants would have missed the opportunity to potentially benefit from treatment.

In other words, Julia's study showed that this advice is probably *wrong*.

Millions of people regularly have blood tests for nutrient deficiency, and most are erroneously told not to take nutrients to treat a mental health condition. Why? Because the belief is that the nutrients can't help them if their blood levels are in the normal range.

Several other studies have shown the same results for overall nutrient levels: they are not helpful at predicting benefit.[2] This is good news — it means that expensive testing is not necessary before trying a broad-spectrum multinutrient treatment. The bad news is that scientists still need to figure out why some people respond to nutrient supplements and some don't.

Blood tests are done on blood drawn from your arm—which does not necessarily reflect what's going on in your brain, or even what your own brain needs.

Julia's lab also looked at this question: Is *change* in a nutrient biomarker correlated with mental health improvement? The overall findings were that they were not.[3] This means that, again, nutrient levels are not helpful at either predicting or monitoring benefit at an individual level. More research is definitely needed.

Why Are Blood Tests Unhelpful?

We used Julia's ADHD study to show you that the nutrient levels detected in your blood tests *do not reliably* predict who could benefit from broad-spectrum supplements.

But some studies have reported on different nutrients and different disorders, with variable results. Rather than focusing on the variability of the scientific data, however, we want to emphasize one incredibly important shortcoming if you are considering getting your blood tested: what is being tested is the circulating level of the nutrient in your body, not your brain. And no test can determine what your brain actually needs.

What About Urine Testing?

As you know by now, *all* the minerals and vitamins are needed for your enzymes to allow for proper brain function. Some people have inherited "sluggish pathways" because their enzymes are *not* efficient, resulting in the need to flood their brains with even more micronutrients than usual. If those enzymes are not working well (for any reason), then the chemicals that should get converted to the next step will accumulate, because the enzymes are not transforming them. Those chemicals have to go somewhere — and that place is your urine, so they can leave your body.

This is why your doctor might suggest an organic acids test, which may be somewhat expensive. The OAT evaluates whether your urine has a lot of those chemicals. If so, then that's an indication that taking a nutrient supplement might improve your enzyme function so you won't have to excrete unused chemicals. In addition, some OAT results can help determine whether you have gut dysbiosis, which you learned about in chapter 3. OAT can also identify yeast (Candida) overgrowth (a common fungal infection). Indeed, Julia had one participant in a clinical study who responded really well to EMP, and two and a half years later she contacted Julia, saying the nutrients were no longer "working." Her psychiatric symptoms had all returned. At the same time, she told Julia that her family physician had diagnosed her with a yeast infection.[4] Treatment of the yeast infection led to improvement in her psychiatric symptoms, suggesting that the yeast problem had interfered with her nutrient absorption — something functional medicine experts have proposed for decades. Although just one case, it illustrated the impact that the onset of a yeast infection can have on recovery.

Are OATs worth the cost? Unfortunately, we can't guide you, because the rationale makes sense, but there hasn't been any independent research on their usefulness for guiding treatment of mental health problems. A significant subset of functional medicine and integrative physicians tell us they find the OAT testing very helpful. The OAT is part of a very new field called metabolomics that is still evolving. Most conventionally trained physicians don't rely on OAT — but most conventional physicians aren't very interested in using nutrients as treatments, either!

Is Deficiency the Right Word?

When discussing nutrient levels, the term "deficiency" can be a problem. First of all, it's inconsistent with how scientists distinguish between "insufficient" levels (meaning a bit low) and a true "deficiency" (which is very low). Studies often show that people with a psychological problem tend, on average, to have nutrient levels lower than those without that problem, but lab testing would still show them as being within the "normal range."[5] Also, the ranges are generally defined as the set of values for 95 percent of the normal population, so they might not be helpful at all for determining what you need for your own *optimal* health.

In other words, you might have a nutrient deficiency *relative to your own metabolic needs* rather than what's considered "normal" for everyone else.

This is why we don't think you should bother with this type of testing. Your emotional status is a better indicator of whether you need a supplement than a blood test is, although monitoring any blood level for safety reasons of course makes perfect sense. Your doctor will help you determine this.

When Blood Testing *Can* Be Helpful

If you have a chronic illness, blood tests are usually part of your regular regimen, and can be very helpful to track how well you're doing. In addition, there are several rare metabolic conditions that can affect your ability to metabolize nutrients:

- Wilson's disease (copper)
- Hemochromatosis (iron)

- Phenylketonuria (phenylalanine)
- Trimethylaminuria (choline)

We detected a case of hemochromatosis during one of our studies, and the participant needed to take a supplement without iron. If you are at risk for these rare conditions, you might want to ask your physician for guidance about testing.

We have also heard some people say they need a test to "prove" they need nutrients. While we understand that having confirmation of a problem might be reassuring to a client, we also want you to know that the tests have not yet been proven to predict response to nutrient treatment.

Finding the Best Mineral and Vitamin Supplements

Figuring out the best supplement might be more complicated than going to outer space! Let us be your guides on your journey. Our advice is *not* about what to take if you are physically unwell, want to optimize your performance training, or are just wondering what to take as "insurance" against future ailments. Our goal is to help anyone struggling with a *mental health problem*. All our advice is grounded in solid scientific evidence.

Bear in mind that other than the B-vitamin formulas, the products tested in research are not usually found over the counter (OTC) except sometimes in health food stores. Most of them are available only through company websites. But the most important thing to know is that the breadth and dose of OTC formulas are usually much smaller than those that have been studied.

Worse, 99 percent of OTC supplements have *never* been tested at all for health benefits! Even fewer have been evaluated by independent scientists — people not biased by any affiliation with the manufacturer. Does that mean these supplements won't help? *We don't know.* If they contain a similar breadth of ingredients to those studied at similar doses, then maybe they will. There are likely to be lots of useful products on the market with lots of anecdotal reports of great benefit. But anecdote is not data. We can't recommend them if there is no published science behind them.

Why Most Companies Don't Want Their Supplements Studied

Although we have made it abundantly clear that we have never had financial ties to any supplement company, Bonnie was still being falsely accused of having a commercial affiliation with the first Alberta supplement company that developed the broad-spectrum multinutrient formula she was studying. She decided to try to do a study that included a product from an American company she had heard good things about, partly so that her reputation would not be so closely tied to the Canadian company. So she phoned the American company, and eventually reached their scientific director. She identified herself and suggested that his company might be interested in some independent science on the usefulness of their supplement for mental health. Dead silence for a few moments.

"Why would we do that?" he eventually replied. "We're making money."

Yes, he really said those exact words.

Julia has also attempted to study other formulas and has been met with a similar level of disinterest. These experiences helped us understand how rare the Alberta supplement companies are, because they devote much time and energy to trying to foster independent scientific research on their products. Most of the research done on other nutrient formulas has had some level of industry financial support.

Breadth and Dose

Before we tell you about what to consider taking, there are two key concepts to understand: *breadth* and *dose*. This information will help you navigate through labels claiming, for example, that they "Contain zinc!" or are "A great source of iron!"

Breadth. In chapter 2, we told you all about the amazing things nutrients do in combination. There is no single magic ingredient to help people feel better; the magic is in the *breadth* of ingredients. As we explained in chapter 1, in all the research on single-nutrient treatments carried out for the last hundred years or so, there have been only modest treatment benefits. We need to consume a broad spectrum of nutrients *in balance* for optimal brain health. So you might wonder just how broad a formula should be.

As you learned in chapter 3, there are approximately fifteen minerals that plants need, and roughly fifteen vitamins that they manufacture. So thirty is a good, basic number.

Notice, however, that thirty refers only to the minerals and vitamins. Many formulas have other types of nutrients as well, such as amino acids, essential fatty acids (e.g., omega-3s), botanicals, and other phytochemicals (e.g., lycopene). So if you're counting up the nutrients in a formula, you need to be careful of what categories you're counting.

We tend to emphasize minerals and vitamins because they are absolutely foundational for good brain function. Omega-3s are also critically important, but because they're difficult to combine with powders or granules, they're rarely packaged together with minerals and vitamins.

Dose. To help you understand dosage, you need to know about Recommended Dietary Allowances, or RDAs.

RDAs were developed during World War II to identify nutritional issues that might "affect national defense." In other words, they were developed to provide adequate nutrient intake for the armed forces.

RDA is currently defined as "the daily dietary intake level of a nutrient considered sufficient by the Food and Nutrition Board of the Institute of Medicine to meet the requirements of 97.5 *percent* of *healthy* individuals in each life-stage and sex group." Note that this means that the numbers are not necessarily adequate for 2.5 percent of the healthy population, and possibly none of the millions of people who have a health challenge.

Consider this another way — the RDAs help identify the *minimum* intake required to avoid a definitive nutritional deficiency, such as scurvy (which can be avoided with just 10 mg of vitamin C). So it is fair to say that RDAs don't come close to identifying what is required for optimal *brain* functioning. As explained in chapter 10, fortification with additional nutrients of many ultra-processed foods (like breakfast cereals) typically provides only small doses of a few nutrients for the purpose of preventing nutritional deficiency diseases.

This is why RDA can't be a useful criterion for people who are suffering from an illness — remember, the values are set for *healthy* individuals. And this is why many of the scientific studies about nutrients use levels above RDA.

Are High Doses Toxic?

We get asked this question all the time.

The rationale for supplementing with nutrient doses higher than the RDA is that some people may have higher nutritional needs than can be provided by food alone. However, higher doses do raise concerns about toxicity, particularly if the dose exceeds the tolerable upper limit (UL). The UL is the maximum daily intake at which adverse health effects are very *unlikely*.

Doesn't that sound contradictory? But it's a crucial point. The UL is *not* identifying when toxicity *will* occur — it's simply that the likelihood of an adverse reaction goes up if what you take exceeds the UL.

As shown in the figure,[6] it's easy to stay below the UL while going above the RDA. Think of that as the *therapeutic window*. The UL is sometimes

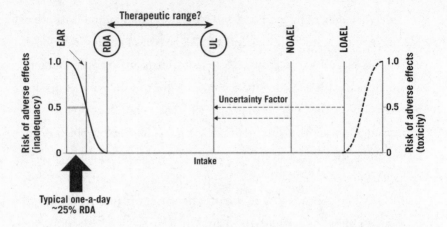

EAR (estimated average requirement) reflects the intake where 50 percent of a population group is at risk of inadequacy. The UL (tolerable upper intake level) is set at an uncertainty factor lower than the NOAEL (no observed adverse effect level) or LOAEL (lowest observed adverse effect level). RDA stands for recommended dietary allowance. From *Food & Nutrition Research* 59, no. 1, under Open Access (CC BY 4.0) from Taylor & Francis Ltd.

ten times higher than the RDA. In other words, you can consume a nutrient way above the RDA without getting anywhere near the UL.

And you won't be surprised to learn that RDAs and ULs are established based on taking a *single nutrient*. Which means it's entirely possible that RDAs and ULs are less relevant when a nutrient is consumed in *combination* with other nutrients. This makes sense, because dietary treatments with single ingredients can actually be harmful. For example, taking folate without vitamin B12 can contribute to masking a B12 deficiency; taking zinc without copper can affect copper metabolism.

So, guess what? To avoid problems, it's best to consume nutrients together, in balance, as nature intended! And in order to obtain a therapeutic effect in *mental health*, you probably need to go over the RDA.

Also please note that the doses for a capsule or pill, which you swallow and then absorb through your gut, may not be the same as the dose

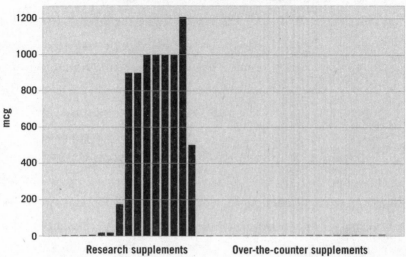

Vitamin B12 Daily Dose in Research Supplements and in Over-the-Counter Supplements

From *New Zealand Journal of Medicine* 127, no. 1395, by permission of New Zealand Medical Association

of a supplement taken a different way, such as with an injection or sublingually. Some companies are working on novel ways to administer the nutrients because some people hate swallowing pills, and the new vehicles they develop for nutrients will affect the therapeutic dose.

Julia supervised a student project relevant to this issue, looking at vitamin doses in children's supplements purchased in supermarkets in New Zealand. This study showed that the doses of OTC products were probably too low to have any effect on mental health symptoms.[7] The graph shows the dramatic difference in a dose of B12 in supplements. Each bar is a different product. On the left are the levels scientists use in their studies; these levels have a proven therapeutic effect on children's mental health. On the right are the supplements sold in the supermarket for kids (like gummies). You can barely see the levels, they are so small! Similar results were found for most of the B vitamins.

Isn't a One-a-Day OTC Supplement Enough?

No, it isn't! Nor should you ever buy a supermarket brand and then just double or triple the dose to attempt to achieve the same doses used in clinical trials. This could lead to consumption of some nutrients at toxic levels, or others too low or out of balance. In the early days of this work, Dr. Charles Popper, a psychiatrist at Harvard, showed that using EMP produced markedly better benefits than OTC pills purchased at a local health food store.[8]

The following list contains all the multinutrient products that we are aware of, for which the cumulative scientific evidence ranging from case studies up to the higher level of evidence from RCTs demonstrates there is potential for improving mental health problems. However, there is no way to predict whether any of these formulas will benefit any particular individual such as yourself or your loved ones.

We have the most detail on the first two formulas on this list, because with more than fifty peer-reviewed studies showing mental health benefits in a variety of experimental designs, they have the strongest scientific base. Future studies are needed to determine whether multinutrients can be used preventatively; to refine dose, delivery and ingredients to maximize clinical response; to explore precise mechanisms of action of the nutrients; and to identify predictors of outcome.

1. For ADHD, mood dysregulation, PMS, symptoms associated with trauma, aggression, depression, stress, anxiety: EMPower™, EMPowerplus™, and EMPowerplus Advanced™ (EMP): www.truehope .com

    For those taking the current EMP formulation for improving mental health symptoms, the dose stipulated on the bottle is two capsules twice a day. However, the dose more typically used in current research is at least four capsules twice a day. For those using these products for assisting with managing stress, our research after

the earthquakes and floods as described in chapter 7 showed that a
therapeutic dose may be lower, such as four a day.

2. For ADHD, smoking cessation, emotional dysregulation, symptoms associated with trauma, aggression, insomnia, stress, anxiety:
Daily Essential Nutrients™ (DEN): www.hardynutritionals.com

A full daily dose for improving psychiatric symptoms with DEN
is four capsules three times a day (twelve/day) and this is the dose
that has been the most used in the cited research. Hardy Nutritionals has a product called Optimal Balance® designed for people just
seeking a little additional nutrient support to manage stress or insomnia. We talked about Optimal Balance in chapters 6 and 7 — Julia used it in the insomnia study as well as following the mosque attacks to help with stress. The typical daily dose is three twice a day
(six/day).

DEN is a better choice than Optimal Balance® for those with
more serious psychiatric problems and/or if taking the nutrients
alongside psychiatric medications, where they may want to consult
with the company product specialists regarding their own situation.

Both DEN and EMP are available as a powder for those who
cannot swallow capsules. Also, some people are very sensitive to the
smell of dietary supplements. If the smell of the capsules is a problem, try keeping them in the fridge or freezer. Pre-pubertal children
may take a lower dose (four twice a day), although we have sometimes gone up to the full adult dose for treating childhood ADHD
in our research. As children enter their teenage years, research has
shown that the dose may need to be increased to maintain symptom control.

Finally, we want to emphasize that the doses mentioned above
are mostly based on our research with people who were *not* taking
any psychiatric medications (e.g., antidepressants, anxiolytics, stimulants) because up to this point, most studies have *excluded* people

taking these meds (the RCTs carried out by Dr. Mehl-Madrona are an exception; see chapter 5).

How Long Do Supplements Take to Work?

Instant improvement is unlikely. Our recommendation based on hundreds of research participants is that you give this treatment at least three months before making a decision on whether it has been helpful for you. Some people may notice benefits within days, others take longer to experience a change. It is hard to predict, although feeling calmer is often one of the first changes people notice.

If you are transitioning from medications to nutrients, psychiatrists' reports indicate you should give it at least six months to a year, as the transition can be challenging (see nutrient/drug information below).

Being consistent and taking all doses is key to optimizing the chances of success.

3. For autism, tantrums, hyperactivity: Brain Child Spectrum Support/ANRC Essentials™: https://www.autismnrc.org

In chapter 5, we told you about several studies conducted by Professor Jim Adams at Arizona State University, using three products: Spectrum Support II/III™, Syndion™, and ANRC Essentials Plus™ (a revised version of Syndion™). Spectrum Support comes as a capsule or colloidal suspension — the standard dose is two capsules (or two teaspoons) twice a day. For ANRC Essentials Plus™, the company provides information on how to gradually increase to the optimal dose based on body weight. The formula comes as either capsules or a powder to mix with your favorite juice (they suggest orange, mango, or cranberry).

4. For stress: Bayer's Berocca™: https://www.buyberocca.com/en/home/

   As discussed in chapter 7, Berocca™ is the most studied formula for reduction of stress. It can be taken as a capsule or an effervescent tablet that you add to water. It has been studied primarily in people drawn from the general population. No concerning side effects have been reported.

5. For stress: Blackmores Executive B™: http://www.blackmores.com.au/products/executive-b-stress-formula

   Blackmores is taken as one capsule twice a day with meals. One study showed improved work-related stress.[9] It is also available as an immediate-release and sustained-release capsule. No side effects have been reported.

6. For stress: Swisse Ultivite™: https://swisse.com/

   Swisse Ultivite™ is available in both a women's and a men's version and is taken as one capsule daily with a meal. Several studies support its use for reduction of stress in otherwise healthy people.[10] No side effects were reported.

7. For aggression in prisoners: Forceval™: www.forceval.co.uk

   Forceval™ is available in a capsule or in effervescent tablets and is a licensed medicine in the United Kingdom. The recommended dose is one capsule daily. The main target for the formula is to combat malnutrition. However, in chapter 6 we described a controlled study using Forceval™ along with fish oil (for omega-3s) to successfully reduce aggression in people incarcerated in prisons. There were no adverse reactions.

8. For depression: Enlyte™: https://www.enlyterx.com/

As mentioned in chapter 5, one study used Enlyte™ to treat people with a variant of the MTHFR gene who also had major depression. The treatment consists of one capsule taken on an empty stomach. It is available by prescription and may be covered by insurance in the United States. Again, no reported side effects.

9. For PMS: Optivite™: www.optimox.com

Optivite™ was first studied in the 1980s and as far as we are aware, there have been no new studies for the last four decades. The product is still available for purchase. The studies we described in chapter 6 suggested between six and twelve capsules a day. The bottle recommends two to six tablets daily with meals. The main concern raised about taking a dose above ten capsules is that it delivers vitamin B6 in a range that can produce some neurological side effects, including tingling of limbs. In Julia's PMS study comparing vitamin B6 to EMP, 25 percent of the women taking B6 reported tingling in their limbs versus 10 percent taking EMP. Fortunately, the side effect is reversible once you stop taking the pills. No participants dropped out of the studies due to side effects.

Do You Gag Just Looking at a Pill?

Many nutrients are available as fairly large capsules, pills, or pressed tablets. When Bonnie first began studying nutrient supplements, she was shocked that some people couldn't participate in her studies because they couldn't swallow the large capsules. She asked one of her students, Roberta Steiger, to research this, and Roberta discovered exactly one article explaining that when we swallow with our head turned slightly to the side, a sphincter muscle in our throat opens a tiny bit wider and stays open a tiny bit longer. That helps with swallowing.

This information led to several studies on the role of head position in swallowing, and then to a training video online that's used around the world (www.research4kids.ucalgary .ca/pillswallowing). Learning different head positions takes a couple weeks of practice with a small candy like TicTacs, although some children learn faster than others. We also have heard that some people benefit from using specialized cups made by companies like Oralflo or GMS.

In the meantime, the delivery systems for multinutrient compounds continue to be improved.

What About Omega-3s?

You learned about the importance of essential fatty acids (EFAs) to the brain and brain development in chapter 2, as well as how crucial it is to try to make sure your diet is rich in omega-3 fatty acids, preferably EPA and DHA, in order to optimize mental health. Omega-3 fatty acids are found at high levels in oily fish and shellfish, plant and nut oils, flaxseed, walnuts, and some algae oils. Some people, however, may not be able to get an adequate supply from their diet and may choose to supplement.

An enormous amount of research has studied omega-3 supplements as treatment for a variety of mental health issues, including bipolar disorder, unstable mood, ADHD, tics, anxiety, and prevention of psychosis. While there are some benefits from fish oil capsules, the effects are sometimes smaller than hoped for, and certainly smaller than what would be expected given the strong correlations observed between fish consumption and mental health (see chapter 4).

For brain health, the greatest amount of positive evidence that has emerged relates to mood disorders and ADHD. For depression, the optimal dose is 1 to 2 g of EPA daily, from either pure EPA or an EPA/DHA (greater than 2:1) formula.[11] Studies at Ohio State University specifically looking at planning and self-regulation in young people with depression or bipolar disorder found that almost two grams (mostly EPA), either alone or in combination with psychotherapy, resulted in greater improvements than psychotherapy did alone.[12]

For ADHD, the optimal dose of EPA should be at least 0.5 g/day.[13] In order to get close to these recommended doses, it's best to take the maximum daily dose recommended on the label (which could be as many as six capsules a day), but even then, many fish oil supplements will not give you the dose that will optimize your chances of improving mood or reducing ADHD symptoms.[14] For some people, these capsules can leave a fishy aftertaste, so you might want to buy a more concentrated formula in order to consume fewer pills.

The most common side effects include stomach upset and fishy taste, but these are minor compared to the proven benefits for expectant mothers, their fetuses, and infants, particularly for neural development. The safe upper limit in pregnancy is unknown.

How can you assess whether a fish oil supplement has adequate amounts of EPA and DHA?

First, you need to know that the amount of EPA+DHA is often quite a bit lower than the amount of total EFAs stated on the bottle. For example, the front of the label might state that each capsule contains 2,000 mg of purified natural fish oil *but* on the back you learn that it only provides 360mg EPA and 240mg DHA. You need to read the entire label to determine the amount of the *active* ingredients. And note that vegetarian sources of EFAs in capsules (like hemp seed or flaxseed) typically have ALA, not DHA and EPA.

However, you don't have to worry about mercury. Julia's lab measured it in ten fish oil products and no trace of it was detected.[15] As many of the companies also make products for the United States, we can feel assured about most US products as well.

What About Herbs, Botanicals, and Single Nutrients for Brain Health?

If you've done any research about nutrients that can improve brain health, you've doubtless seen information about herbs and botanicals. The reason we're not covering them in this book is that scientists still don't know exactly *how* they influence brain health. In contrast to minerals and vitamins, which we know humans have evolved to need, it just is not clear whether botanicals are essential for a healthy brain. We recognize that benefits have been reported from botanicals like St John's wort, kava kava, passionflower, curcumin, lemon balm, ashwagandha, lavender, saffron, sage, and ginkgo, but more research needs to be done to define the mechanism by which they improve brain function. Until that happens, botanicals are not classified as being essential for mental or physical health, even though there are many known to be useful for their antioxidant and anti-inflammatory properties.

There are also some individual nutrients that have had varying success for the treatment of mental health problems, like NAC, SAMe, zinc, magnesium, and vitamin D. We are deliberately staying away from reviewing these single-nutrient approaches as they do not conform to the biology that we described in detail in chapter 2. They may well help offer relief to some individuals on their own for certain conditions, but

based on human physiology, we expect that people are likely
to get much more powerful effects with a broad combination
formula.

Pros and Cons: Nutrients Won't Kill You — But Prescription Pharmaceuticals Certainly Can

Prescription medications save lives and solve health problems for many, but may also cause hundreds of thousands of deaths every year. Many of these deaths are a direct result of the over-prescription of addictive opioids. But long-term use of psychiatric medications has also been associated with early death.

The CDC reported in 2011 on death rates from prescription medication, as follows: "The United States is in the grip of an epidemic of prescription drug overdoses. Over 27,000 people died from overdoses in 2007, a number that has risen fivefold since 1990 and has never been higher. Prescription drugs are now involved in more overdose deaths than heroin and cocaine combined."

Data from over thirty years in the United States showed that adverse drug reactions for all meds were between the fourth and sixth leading cause of death in America, and serious ADRs from psychiatric medications were disproportionately high relative to other medications.[16]

Another concerning trend is some recent data on medication-induced loss of brain cells. In 2020, a blinded, placebo-controlled trial of a popular antipsychotic medication (Zyprexa, or olanzapine) demonstrated decreased thickness of the cortex in the brains of people who took it.[17]

Bottom line: even when used properly and accurately, medications, especially psychiatric medications, may be a significant cause of death in America. Their impact on brain structure is a topic needing much more research.[18] What about nutrients? In Canada, no one has died from improving their diet or from taking a nutrient supplement since the country began keeping records in 1967. And in America, according to the 2017 Annual Report of the American Association of Poison Control Center, no one has ever died from a vitamin pill.[19]

Are You Just Peeing Away Your Money?

Critics of nutrient supplements are quick to accuse us of giving patients expensive urine. In other words, they believe the micronutrients will just be excreted because you don't need them. Well, you know by now, thanks to all the research you've already read about in this book, that this is just not true. When people with a psychological problem take nutrients, their brains and bodies *do* use them! They *do* change biological function — like gene expression, brain function, and the diversity of the bacteria in your gut microbiome.[20]

An even more disheartening accusation comes routinely from medical professionals who should know better. "My psychiatrist said there is no evidence that nutrient treatment helps with mental health" is something we hear all the time. What we think these psychiatrists *mean* is that nutrient treatments are not part of the clinical practice guidelines (CPGs) and therefore cannot possibly be effective. And as we explained in chapter 1, CPGs are written by committees often dominated by individuals funded by pharmaceutical companies,[21] so we do not expect these guidelines to mention nutrients for the foreseeable future.

If you hear a statement like the one above, it means your psychiatrist hasn't read the scientific literature that details all the studies you've read about in this book, and more! As you know by now, we are strong supporters of evidence-based treatments, and the science behind using nutrients and nutrition to prevent and/or treat mental disorders is very real and very well proven.

We are also troubled by authors not distinguishing between physical and mental health. For example, in his book *Killing Us Softly*, Dr. Paul Offit criticizes various alternative health approaches such as homeopathy and Chinese herbs, and dismisses all nutrient supplements for the treatment of any illness — but *he doesn't even mention* mental illness! Yet his book is often used as evidence against nutrients for the treatment of mental health challenges.

Are There Side Effects from Broad-Spectrum Multinutrient Supplements?

So far, none of the broad-spectrum multinutrient formulas or the B-complex formulas have produced any serious adverse effects. This information is, however, based on studies conducted with people *not concurrently taking psychiatric medications* (see "Nutrient/Drug Interactions" later in this chapter).

The most common side effects reported are headaches, dry mouth, rash, and stomachaches, although they are typically mild, transitory, and can be avoided by taking capsules on a full stomach and with plenty of water. These side effects do not occur more frequently than in those taking a placebo. And as you have learned, people report a number of positive "side effects," such as relief of constipation, improved sleep, and more energy.

A minority of participants report feeling more agitated, possibly due to the dose being too high for them; lowering the dose tends to fix this. The dropout rate due to side effects across our research has been very low (about 5 percent, with no difference between the active and placebo groups). Our overall dropout rate is typically 10–15 percent. It is challenging to compare this rate to psychiatric drugs, because it is not always known why people drop out. A recent systematic review of seventy-three placebo-controlled trials of antidepressants found, however, that at least two and a half times as many people dropped out, a rate that can be as high as 75 percent, due to adverse events compared to those receiving a placebo.[22] These comparisons suggest that nutrients are causing fewer intolerable side effects as compared with medications.

Are Broad-Spectrum Multinutrients Really Safe?

Remember that we pointed out that supplementation with single ingredients can actually be harmful. As Dr. Bryan Kolb, a Canadian neuroscientist, explained, "Supplementation with a large dose of only one nutrient could skew affiliated biochemical cascades."[23] But the fact that the multinutrient formulas are broad-spectrum and balanced does not prove they are safe. Fortunately, a lot of safety information has been published on them.

Many of the studies conducted on EMP and DEN collected safety data (via blood tests) before and after exposure to the nutrients, typically over two or three months. This means the researchers looked at markers such as kidney and liver functioning before and after the participants took the nutrients. Some of the studies have also compared those results with people taking a placebo to control for the passage of time or time of year. In all of these studies, amounting to several hundred blood tests done before and at the end of the studies, no evidence of clinically meaningful short-term harm was seen. This does not prove that no one will ever have a serious ADR, but it has not happened in twenty years of research.

In addition, people experience less discomfort from multinutrient treatment. In the study described in chapter 5, the forty-four people with autism taking prescription meds experienced ten times as many ADRs as the forty-four people with autism taking broad-spectrum multinutrients.

Occasionally, a blood marker rose while remaining within the normal range but the change has not been found in longer trials, meaning that the observation was probably spurious. Bonnie and her colleagues collated data from 144 children and adults participating in six different studies and found no significant adverse effects.[24] Safety of ANRC Essentials

Plus™ over a one-year period found no health concerns in their extensive blood testing panel.[25]

In 2019 Julia's lab looked at *long-term* exposure to the multinutrients in people who had taken one of the Alberta formulas for one to twelve years (the average was just over three years).[26] Out of approximately 1,000 assays, 5 percent of the blood tests were outside the reference range, exactly what would be expected by chance alone with any sampling method. Also, there was no recurring pattern of change indicative of a specific negative effect.

The researchers also asked about side effects from taking the nutrients long term and none were reported. Based on over 200 research participants, Julia has learned that the primary drivers for stopping the nutrients were the cost and the number of pills to swallow.

The follow-up information enabled us to answer a critical question about long-term efficacy. Based on psychological questionnaires, about 85 percent of former research participants are in remission long term. Contrast that to research on antidepressants that shows only about a quarter of people go into remission long term.[27] It is gratifying to show that taking nutrients long term has real results.

Are we saying the nutrients are absolutely safe for you? No one can ever guarantee *100 percent* safety for anything! But what we can say is that there's nothing to suggest that nutrients are unsafe when consumed together, in balance.

Also, remember, we are not recommending these nutrients for people who do *not* have mental health issues. In those cases, it is likely that a much lower dose would be useful. Our research is based on people trying to resolve psychological problems. You always need to consider the potential benefit of reducing or eliminating your symptoms (alongside minimal or no side effects) compared to the very low possibility of long-term harm.

There is one other question we often hear: "Will the nutrients stop working for me?" This is a perfectly understandable question from people who've already had that experience with a psychiatric medication. Fortunately, there is no habituation to the nutrients — in fact, if humans habituated to nutrients, our species would have become extinct long ago!

But there is one interesting phenomenon that is very reassuring: over time, many people can decrease their dose. This is likely because they've refilled their bodily storage depots for these nutrients. Most people are also sensitive enough to how good or bad they're feeling so that they can adjust their dose for any current situation. Are exams or a huge project at work approaching or are you feeling a little under the weather? Help mitigate the stress or support your immune system by increasing your dose. Are you going through a growth spurt or experiencing PMS? Increase the dose temporarily. Life is going along pretty smoothly? Maybe lower the dose a bit if you can.

If you're worried, there's no harm in having routine blood tests, and obviously it makes good sense to get any new symptoms checked out. The physicians we work with on our studies recommend that people have a routine screening for metabolic and electrolyte abnormalities before they begin their new regimen, and intermittently during follow-up.[28]

The Difference Between a Health Claim and a Therapeutic Claim

One significant problem with taking nutrients to treat any health problem is that by law, manufacturers are prohibited from listing any therapeutic benefits on labels even where there is strong scientific support for it. This is shocking, even ludicrous!

This law is in place because supplements are generally classified as foods, not medicines, so the label can't specify a *therapeutic claim*. A therapeutic claim refers to preventing, alleviating, curing, and treating diseases, ailments, defects, and injuries. They are reserved for medicines

All the scaremongering about how supplements are dangerous or killing us is based on single-nutrient studies of physical—not mental—health applications, but it reinforces physicians and the public to ignore the burgeoning research in this field.

only. This is ridiculous, when you think about it. Don't we learn as children that eating carrots prevents deterioration in vision? But a carrot farmer would not be allowed to state that on a bag of carrots.

In contrast, supplements are limited to claims of a *health benefit,* which is generally limited to the maintenance or promotion of health or wellness. A health claim can't state that it's a treatment or cure for an ailment.

For example, a therapeutic claim — which can never appear on a bottle of nutrients no matter how many published studies there are — would be "Treats or cures mood disorders." On the other hand, an allowable health claim is "Enhances mental well-being." Or "Supports wellness." Or "Improves brain health."

What about the other side of the coin: Should nutrient supplements be required to show a health benefit before they can be sold? Since the vast majority of formulas are unstudied, that would remove most of them from the shelves.

There are no easy answers, but we do know that our current system — where you have no idea if your OTC supplement has been scientifically proven to improve mental health symptoms — needs to change.

Ignore the Critics!

What if you're feeling better from taking nutrients to improve your mental health—but then you see headlines like: "Your

Vitamins Are Killing You!" or "The Dark Side of Antioxidants!" Should you worry?

Over a decade ago, a massive amount of media attention focused on a meta-analysis of antioxidant supplements for prevention of death, published by researchers from the University of Nis in Serbia.[29] The authors concluded that vitamin A, beta carotene, and vitamin E may increase the death rate.

There was a huge amount of criticism on how these authors analyzed their data, especially as the difference in mortality between the groups of people taking antioxidants (13.1 percent) versus those not taking them (10.5 percent) was very small. Also, this study didn't even report if those people died *because* of the supplements. Surely some died from accidents or long-term illnesses. This is another example of *correlation doesn't prove causation.*

A few years later, researchers from the University of Hohenheim in Germany used the same data and came to a different conclusion—showing that there were far more health benefits for those who took the supplements.[30] Again, they looked only at physical health, and reported that 36 percent of the studies showed that antioxidant supplements resulted in a positive health outcome; 60 percent of the studies showed no effect; and only 4 percent had negative results.

Research studies that show no benefit to mortality or heart disease should not have their results extrapolated to *mental* health. Obviously, some people might not ever benefit from supplements. But the vulnerable portion of our population—those with mental challenges, the poor, and those who do not have good access to nutritious food—are very likely to benefit.

Nutrient/Drug Interactions

It is important, of course, to know that certain supplements and foods can interact with certain prescription medications and cause side effects.

Do Nutrients Amplify Medication Effects?

We need to talk a bit about a philosophical issue. A number of studies as early as 1992 showed that giving a few vitamins to patients on antidepressants resulted in them being able to lower their medications.[31] Bonnie remembers seeing an issue of the *Harvard Mental Health Letter* dated October 2008, entitled "Herbal and Dietary Supplements for Depression," and thinking "At last! Some people are starting to realize that nutrient treatment of psychiatric symptoms is possible!" But the excitement turned to disappointment when the article turned out to be evaluating nutrients to "boost" the impact of psychiatric medications. In other words, the nutrients were seen *only* as useful helpers to prescription meds. Not, obviously, as a possible replacement.

Clearly, the two of us are not on the same wavelength with the philosophy that *boosting* the impact of psych meds is the primary goal of nutrient supplementation!

Is this an important difference?

Combining psychiatric meds with the broad-spectrum multinutrient formulas is probably one of the most challenging aspects of this work. Physicians regularly report that side effects increase when their patients start adding nutrients to their psychiatric medications, a phenomenon sometimes interpreted as the nutrients amplifying the effect of the medications.[32]

One of the studies of ANRC Essentials Plus™ involving children and adults with autism also reported this phenomenon. About a third of the people were on medications (like antipsychotics), and that subgroup had less improvement from the nutrients than those not taking medications.

These observations may be puzzling for some physicians, given their expectation that nutrients shouldn't interfere with prescription meds. But they shouldn't be puzzled, because the ability to lower medication dose when adding nutrient supplements has been known for so long.[33]

This suggests what we call the dark side of using nutrients to boost the effect of psychiatric medication. Is there a bright side? We think there is.

Back in 2001, Dr. Charles Popper wrote a commentary on one of Bonnie's earliest studies that showed how beneficial a broad-spectrum multinutrient formula was for fourteen adults with bipolar disorder.[34] Most of the patients were able to reduce their meds, some becoming stable with no meds at all. Popper used the same formula in his clinical case series — nineteen of his twenty-two patients showed a positive response — and then he addressed how the nutrients interacted with their psych meds. The term he used was *potentiation* — the multinutrient formula seemed to *potentiate* the effect of prescribed psychiatric medications.

The solution was simple, though counterintuitive to some: reduce or eliminate the meds after introducing the nutrients. This is often referred to as a *cross-titration*. You begin the nutrients, and as you gradually increase the dose, you also begin to gradually decrease the meds.[35]

Potentiation is good news! It allows people to lower their psychiatric meds while replacing them with nutrients that are safe and free of significant side effects.

Bonnie proved this in 2009 when, along with Professor Dermot Gately from New York University, she published a database analysis on bipolar disorder. The data were drawn from 358 adults who took EMP and tracked their symptoms for a minimum of six months.[36] The people who did cross-titrations, reducing their medications as they increased their nutrients, benefited far more than the people who continued taking their higher doses of medications. In other words, *not* lowering meds prevents the optimum benefit from nutrient treatments. We've observed the same patterns in children as well.[37]

While it's okay to think of nutrients as a way to boost the efficacy of medications, also think of them as a way to *reduce and/or replace* those medications. Here's why:

Brain Function

You've learned already that the neurotransmitters in your brain go through many metabolic steps involving their synthesis, uptake, and breakdown. Each of those steps requires enzymes, and every enzyme is dependent upon multiple cofactors, which include a variety of vitamins and minerals. If the multinutrient treatment provides enough minerals and vitamins so that even enzymes with drastically reduced activity become so supersaturated with the necessary cofactors, then near-normal function may be restored. When this happens, medication would no longer be necessary for those functions.

Liver Function

Has your physician ever told you not to eat grapefruit or drink grapefruit juice while taking a certain medication? The reason is very simple. Medications are broken down in your liver and small intestine by a specialized group of enzymes called cytochrome P450 (CYPs). Grapefruit interferes with this process by blocking CYPs. In fact, studies show that grapefruit and some other citrus fruits block CYPs so effectively that they increase the blood levels of over *eighty-five different* medications, which can then increase their side effects.[38] Even small amounts of grapefruit can cause severe problems with certain drugs.

A similar process might occur when you take nutrients along with psychiatric meds. Nutrients such as vitamin D and niacin can inhibit various CYP enzymes, changing the rate of medication breakdown, similar to the action of grapefruit.

Does this mean you should stop eating food that contains vitamins and minerals? Of course not. But more research is needed to guide physicians on nutrient/drug interactions and the best way to cross-titrate. In the meantime, we advise caution when combining nutrients with psychiatric medications you are already taking. Your recovery may be slower and more difficult compared to people who are unmedicated.

When you want to start taking nutrients, it is absolutely crucial that you *do not stop* taking the meds for your psychiatric condition. We suggest you discuss options with your prescribing physician first. If that individual is not knowledgeable about nutrients, or not open to nutritional treatments, you may need to look elsewhere for support and consultation. If you want to do a cross-titration, call one of the supplement companies and discuss it with one of their product specialists. They are trained for this exact purpose, and are available to liaise with health professionals in your life.

You might also find it helpful to bring along the references listed for chapters 5 through 7 when you're discussing your options with your prescribing physician — or even better, give your doctor a copy of this book! Many physicians are *not* familiar with multinutrient treatment, and hopefully what you've learned in this book will help you override any skepticism.

Some people find the transition to nutrients is difficult, while others sail through with no hint of any problems. At this time, it's impossible to predict who might have any issues and who won't, just as we can't predict who will benefit from a broad-spectrum multinutrient formula or not.

Other Medication Interactions

One other type of medication interaction is worth noting. As you learned in previous chapters, having a healthy intestinal microbiome is very important, especially for the proper absorption of the nutrients in your food. But sometimes you must take an antibiotic due to a physical health condition, and it can cause an imbalance of the normal communities of microorganisms that live inside you. When that happens, micronutrient supplements (as well as the nutrients from your diet) may not be absorbed as well as usual. Some people have reported that they find it is very helpful to increase their multinutrient dose alongside the antibiotic during that period of time. Probiotics have also been shown to be helpful to assist with healing gastrointestinal problems and promoting better nutrient absorption.[39]

The Takeaway

1. The long-term follow-up of research participants from Julia's lab has shown that ongoing treatment with broad-spectrum multinutrients results in 80 to 85 percent going into remission from their mental health symptoms. In contrast, a more typical long-term remission rate for those taking antidepressant meds is less than 25 percent.

2. Blood testing may be important to consider for general health and safety, and we encourage you to discuss your specific needs with your healthcare provider. But levels of nutrients measured from standard blood tests have not been shown to *predict* whether you will feel better after taking a broad-spectrum formula.

3. The published safety and toxicity data for broad-spectrum multinutrient treatment are very reassuring. Minor problems such as initial nausea can usually be handled by taking the capsules on a full stomach with lots of water, and no significant adverse side effects have been reported even after long-term use.

4. The vast majority of the studies carried out on the broad-spectrum formulas has required that people be unmedicated

at the time of the study. Clinically, we know that significant adverse events can happen to people taking psychiatric meds who are not guided in a cross-titration (gradually increasing nutrients, and then tapering down meds). If your physician is not knowledgeable on cross-titration, the product specialists at the Alberta supplement companies offer this guidance. They also offer training to physicians on how to do this safely.

5. A big challenge for consumers is that evidence-based use — such as a multinutrient supplement to treat mood problems — is not permitted to be stated on the labels of natural health products. Manufacturers can only make limited health claims such as "enhances well-being."

12

A VISION FOR A HAPPIER, HEALTHIER TOMORROW

We are never 100 percent sure about anything . . . We shouldn't be looking for certainty; instead we need to be saying to ourselves, when do we have enough evidence to make good decisions?

— PROFESSOR CAILIN O'CONNOR,
WHEN TALKING ABOUT HER BOOK, *The Misinformation Age*

ACCLAIMED SCIENCE FICTION AUTHOR Sir Arthur Clarke wrote that all new ideas pass through three periods, consistent with the three stages defined by Schopenhauer we described in the Introduction:

1. It can't be true.
2. It's probably true but not important.
3. I knew all along it was a good idea!

This is why we've written this book, because we hope it will move our society closer to recognizing that nutrient prevention and treatment for mental health issues are more than just a good idea — they can be life-savers.

What If . . . Nutrition Could Treat Mental Illness?

The question is, has our society reached the point of recognizing nutrition as a critical player in the resolution of this terrible epidemic of mental health challenges? In other words, what if everything you have read in this book is true? What ought to happen next?

Malcolm Gladwell popularized the notion of a tipping point in his best-seller of the same name, describing how ideas, products, messages, and behaviors can suddenly spread quickly. That unique tipping point happens when an idea becomes contagious; change no longer comes about gradually, but at one dramatic moment. Could we be close to reaching that tipping point for nutrition and mental health?

There are moments when we despair, especially when it seems that brain health is being excluded from so many discussions of diet and health. For instance, in May 2019, a major medical journal, the *Lancet,* published "Health Effects of Dietary Risks in 195 countries 1990–2017," and mental health *was not mentioned even once.* Cancer, heart disease, shortened lifespans, diabetes — these are all very important health matters. But as you learned in chapter 2, it is our brains that absorb and utilize a disproportionately large amount of the nutrients we consume. A consideration of the health effects from dietary factors that excludes brain and mental health is missing a very big point!

That's why Bonnie calls many of her lectures "Nutrition Above the Neck" — to focus people on the fact that the brain is neglected much too often in discussions about nutrition.

An editorial a few years ago in the *Annals of Internal Medicine* was entitled "Enough Is Enough: Stop Wasting Money on Vitamin and Mineral Supplements."[1] They were referring to studies in physical health that used one or two selected nutrients. The title of that article should have been: "Enough Is Enough: Stop Wasting Money on Magic Bullet Research on

Single Nutrients for Physical Health!" All of these vocal critics and their misleading titles do a grave disservice to the rigorous and well-conducted research showing all the benefits of additional nutrients for people with mental health issues.

Even within a government agency focused on dietary supplements, mental health seems to be relatively neglected. A recent analysis of US funding for dietary supplements through the National Institutes of Health reported that the Office of Dietary Supplements supported studies primarily with the following three outcome issues: cancer, cardiovascular disease, and women's reproductive health.[2] But what about *mental* health?

There are also some bright moments, fortunately, such as the one in November 2019 when, for the first time that we know of, a major American network (CBS) carried a brief segment on nutrition and mental health in their program *Sunday Morning.* Or the cover story in the March 2020 edition of *Oprah* magazine entitled "New Science on Food That'll Change Your Mood." Or when our earthquake and flood studies were featured in the UK newspaper the *Guardian* in February 2020 on nutrition post-trauma. Or when we get recognized with awards for the work that we do. All of these examples demonstrate that the public is beginning to hear the message that nutrition is important for mental health.

Our Vision: As Easy as One, Two, Three

People sometimes ask us why we keep studying nutrients in pill form while at the same time emphasizing overall dietary intake in our lectures (and in this book!). First, our studies of nutrients in capsules are really a *proof of principle.* The fact is, we cannot put the whole world on pills, although pharmaceutical companies seem to have that goal! Doing studies using nutrients in capsules has enabled us to demonstrate the importance of minerals and vitamins for mental health in many of the people you have read about throughout this book. By conducting studies with a variety of designs, including comparing the nutrients to placebo, we can robustly argue against the critics who say it is all just a big placebo effect.

Nutrients in capsules play a second really critical role: they enable people who seem to have a predisposition to require an unusually large amount of nutrients — more than they can get from their food — to experience the benefits of good nutrition. For many people, additional nutrients make all the difference.

The ideal treatment paradigm in our Vision for a Happier, Healthier Tomorrow takes mental health care through three steps:

Step One in Our Vision for the Future. People struggling with mental health challenges will be educated by every single mental health clinic about eating only real food, and how it will save them money and improve their health. They'll also be guided about shopping — what you learned about purging your pantry, planning your grocery list, buying your food, and cooking for a whole foods Mediterranean type of diet.

Ideally, this education would also be directed to college students. All over the world, university counseling centers are reporting an enormous surge in referrals. Some report that over half of their entire student body passes through their doors during their undergraduate years. At all levels, there seems to be an escalating rate of suicides, drug dependence, and sick leave for mental health treatment and recovery.

Yet despite all the evidence described in this book, when the August 2019 issue of *Nature* published a description of a new, large, well-funded investigation into the mental health of American graduate students, entitled "A Better Future for Graduate-Student Mental Health," there was not one single word in it about nutrition or diet . . . despite the fact that the subtitle was "A Consortium of US Universities Aims to Examine How Best to Help a Vulnerable Population That Is Affected by Anxiety and Depression."

College Students Need to Eat Better—
Who's Going to Tell Them?

What do college students eat? The first words that probably popped into your mind are pizza, soda, beer, and ramen! Now, ask a few college students you know to write down everything they eat or drink for two days. When you see their lists, are you going to be handing them this book and urging them to read it? We hope so. College students are living with intense stress and pressure to succeed. They are in dire need of all the brain power they can get to do well in their studies. Let's help them eat better.

Step Two in Our Vision. People who don't get enough benefit from improving their diet will be encouraged to take a broad-spectrum multinutrient formula giving them all the major minerals and vitamins in balance, plus appropriate amounts and sources of omega-3s.

As you learned in chapter 11, the vast majority of the OTC multinutrient products have trivial amounts of vitamins and few minerals. That doesn't make them bad — just not enough. When taken in balance, vitamins and minerals are not going to harm or kill you. There is a very large window of safety between supplements with low RDA levels, and the much higher cutoff where safety concerns arise. Multinutrient products all fall within that safe window.

Step Three in Our Vision. People who aren't benefiting from Step One (diet education and improvements) plus Step Two (nutrient supplementation) will be referred for further counseling, possible medication, and/or family therapy.

You may wonder why we don't suggest counseling and family therapy earlier, perhaps in Step One or Two. The reason is that we've been told so very often by people that they were not able to absorb and/or implement strategies taught in therapy until *after* their thoughts had cleared following better nutrition. Many have said that they would have benefited from all other treatments to a much greater extent if someone had taught them to improve nutrient intake *first*, with diet and/or broad-spectrum supplementation.

Notice also that we don't say, "Never take psychiatric medications." Denying that some people benefit from psychiatric medication at certain times is just as narrow-minded as denying that nutrients help sustain healthy brain activity.

Knowing that "pre-treatment" with nutrition and supplements helps with resilience and clearing people's brain fog is why we urge mental health clinics to *begin all new referrals* by educating about nutrition and mental health, teaching them to shop for whole foods, and even holding cooking classes. Based on the studies we described in chapter 4, we'd predict that *at least* one-third of their referrals will no longer need additional mental health care. Given that all our mental health resources are stretched very thin, isn't this a good-news story?

In other words, in our Vision for a Happier, Healthier Tomorrow, nutrition will be the *primary treatment* that patients get *first*; medication will be considered a *supplement* if it is needed at all. That's why it's sometimes difficult for us to refer to pill-form nutrients as supplements — for us, they're primary treatments!

Each of Us Is Unique

In chapter 6 we cited some information from the 1956 book by biochemist Roger Williams entitled *Biochemical Individuality*. In twenty normal, healthy men, the variability in their body chemistry was remarkable. For instance, there was a sixfold difference in calcium levels in the urine between two individuals; others had a threefold variation in their blood levels of magnesium.

Until personalized testing becomes more advanced, what you can easily do right now is improve your nutrient intake, and — if you choose to take a multinutrient supplement — know that there's no apparent harm in doing so if you are not currently taking a psychiatric medication. If you *are* currently taking medication, you should consult your prescribing physician and reread the section on nutrient/drug interactions in chapter 11.

Each of Us Is Complicated

Nutrition is not an isolated variable. It is normal to find that good nutrition correlates with exercise, for example, because people who are conscious of their health pay attention to both, and together, they can have a major impact. The Furukawa Nutrition and Health study published in 2019 found that poor diet and low amounts of exercise combined were a powerful predictor of the emergence of depression symptoms.[3]

Over time, people tend to figure out that there are many factors affecting their mental well-being. As Dr. Andrew Weil points out in his book *Spontaneous Happiness,* there are some basic principles to keep in mind: "It is normal and healthy to experience a variable range of moods and emotions both positive and negative . . . [and] . . . It is unrealistic to be happy all the time." Accepting such principles is important. Also, doing what your parents and grandparents probably told you is a pretty good idea: eat right, sleep right, and everything in moderation. Your social network and community ties should also be pillars of your emotional well-being.

Knowledge Is Power

Knowledge influences changes in health behavior. Smoking was once considered to be just a bad habit until we realized that nicotine is an addictive drug, other chemicals in cigarettes are carcinogenic, and people were dying as a result.

But the real tipping point for change came when secondhand smoke was shown to harm nonsmokers. It became unacceptable to expose family and friends to cigarette smoke, and regulations and laws soon followed. In other words, social change emerged when it was understood that smoking was more than a personal choice or a habit: it was an addiction that imposed a societal burden, and changes needed to be made or everyone's health was at risk.

The plague of increasing mental health issues needs to be treated the same way. What people eat has societal implications because of the tremendous impact on entire families and on healthcare budgets.

How do we get to that point? As with so much in life, the path forward depends on education.

Improve Nutrition Education from a Young Age

Whenever possible, both of us have been teaching some basics about brain metabolism to teachers, school staff, and children as young as eleven. Inevitably, the one thing people seem to particularly appreciate is the diagram of the piece of serotonin pathway we showed you in chapter 2. This response has been going on for about a decade, so we both almost always use that diagram in every one of our lectures, no matter who's in the audience, or how educated they are. It's that light bulb moment where everyone goes, "Oh, so that's *why* I should eat healthy!"

The several studies we reviewed in chapter 4 where people were taught about a whole food, Mediterranean-style diet all showed that people *did* improve their diet and *did* experience improved mental health. The sooner children learn this, the sooner their parents will learn it, too. Isn't it time to begin teaching this in elementary school, before many more children experience depression and anxiety?

The Role of Nutrients in Brain Function Should Be Taught to All Physicians and Other Clinicians

Despite the wealth of knowledge linking food and health, nutrition receives little attention in medical practice.[4] As you know by now, this is mostly due to the severe deficiency of nutrition education at all levels of medical training.

The opposition we often encounter from psychiatrists toward the use of nutrient treatment stems from their lack of education. The story of Ginger in chapter 5 was clear evidence of how a psychiatrist's ignorance (and fear!) can block progress in this field. This email, sent to Bonnie in 2001, echoes Ginger's ordeal:

> My daughter has been taking the EMP supplement for the past three months. I cannot believe the difference this has made in her life. She is able to concentrate (before, she could not remember things and was unable to study) and she is not feeling depressed. Taking EMP has given her back her life. We are very grateful to her counselor, who has spent many hours on the phone giving us excellent advice. She deserves a medal. I am sorry that my daughter's psychiatrist has not been supportive of her decision to take EMP. My daughter really feels abandoned by the medical profession.

When a Doctor Really Gets It

In chapter 1 we introduced you to Andrew, whose psychosis was "fixed" with one of the Alberta formulas. We described the long-term impact on him and his family, and also the cost savings. But what about his psychiatrist, Dr. Rodway?

When Bonnie first encountered Dr. Rodway in 2008, at the end of the meeting with Andrew's parents, she invited Bonnie into her office and immediately said, "I am this close [indicating a tiny gap with her fingers] to stopping prescribing these drugs for children." But what choice did she have? She could have reacted like Ginger's psychiatrist (shutting the door and her mind), but she did not.

Andrew's subsequent response to the nutrients caused Dr. Rodway to re-evaluate her choices for treating patients. She enrolled in the two-year Fellowship Program in Integrative Medicine created by Dr. Andrew Weil at the University of Arizona and left her clinical position. She is now an integrative psychiatrist in private practice, with the freedom to treat her patients with non-pharmaceutical treatments *first* (though not necessarily exclusively). She describes her current clinical practice this way: "I start with the 'foundations' of eating well, exercising to the best of one's ability, employing evidence-based sleep hygiene tools, regularly practicing breath work, experimenting with and then finding the discipline to practice a comfortable style of daily meditation and, finally, encouraging psycho-spiritual growth."

This is the education needed for clinicians, so that their knee-jerk response to any questions about non-drug alternatives is not "there is no evidence" — even when there often is.

The Impact on Our Society of the Future

Two one-year follow-up studies from Julia's lab showed that people often stop taking their nutrients even when they had successfully treated challenging psychiatric symptoms and they felt so much better. Why? The cost. Supplements aren't yet covered by insurance and high-quality supplements can be expensive. Patients who can't afford them often switch back to their meds — even knowing how debilitating the side effects can be — because the cost for the meds is subsidized or covered by insurance. The issue isn't that there's no funding available to pay for nutrient treatment — it's just that this funding needs to be redirected within a system that is no longer driven largely by the pharmaceutical industry.

In Alberta, Bonnie and others have tried for years to get the provincial healthcare system to put multinutrient supplements on the approved list that would enable doctors to prescribe them for mental health and for patients to obtain them at little or no cost. Julia has repeatedly tried the same thing in New Zealand and continues to be turned down, usually justified with a standard response of "there is simply not enough evidence." To the best of our knowledge, there is no insurance system in the United States that will cover the cost of a nutrient formula for mental health, although there are some individual nutrients, such as folic acid, that are covered for heart health or prenatal use. *People should be able to afford better food and nutrient supplements for optimal mental health.*

Based on how many phone calls, emails, and invitations to speak we've both received for many years, we believe that the public *is* ready to accept the importance of nutrition for mental health. What could happen if the policy makers finally begin to pay attention and help us move to our Happier, Healthier Tomorrow?

We are aware of insurance companies that are rewarding their customers for making healthier food choices at the supermarket by lowering their premiums. Other insurance companies recognize the value of insuring clients who actively participate in healthy lifestyle behaviors. Just like smoking increases your premiums, should eating ultra-processed food carry the same penalty? When society realizes that ultra-processed is not a necessity of life, perhaps that might happen.

Money is a great motivator!

There Will Be Massive Savings for Our Healthcare Budgets

In two extensively documented case studies, Bonnie and her colleagues have shown that treatment with broad-spectrum multinutrients not only resolved the mental health problems, but also they cost *less than 10 percent of conventional care.* One of those cases was Andrew (see chapter 1), and the other was Marie.

Over a decade ago, Bonnie met a woman in her forties who described how she had recovered from severe psychiatric problems by taking EMP. We both hear these stories so often but they continue to amaze us. But what Marie said next had an even bigger impact: "You know, you really should pull all my health records and analyze what my mental health treatment cost the government. It must have been more than a million dollars. And now I need no mental health services at all."

Marie was first treated in 1997 in Ontario when she was thirty-three. Her diagnoses over the next four years included bipolar disorder with psychotic symptoms, schizoaffective disorder, depression, and post-traumatic stress disorder. She was in and out of hospitals in three provinces until December 2001. Marie herself estimates she was an inpatient about 70 percent of the time.

Bonnie knew we were years away from doing a proper large-group evaluation of cost savings of multinutrient treatments, but we have a single-payer system in Canada, so she wondered if it would be worth retrieving that information for a single case. Bonnie approached two University of Toronto health economists who thought it was possible if we requested only inpatient costs, because it would have been too difficult to obtain all the records for all of Marie's outpatient psychiatric appointments and medications. It still took over a year for us to get the information we needed to publish the amazing results.[5]

The average annual inpatient cost for those five years of conventional psychiatric care was about $60,000 in Canadian dollars. On December 1, 2001, Marie began taking EMP. She has never needed any additional mental health care — no doctor's appointments, no medication, no outpatient therapy. A psychiatrist described her use of the multinutrient formula this way: "It is probably true that it is the most effective single treatment which [Marie] has tried." Her choice of treatment translates to a cost saving of $60,000 times twenty years — or *$1.2 million,* for inpatient treatment alone. This figure is clearly a gross underestimate of the total cost savings — since it excludes clinic visits — and this represents just one individual!

Marie currently has to spend about $720/year for her nutrients, because even though the government is saving a minimum estimated projection of $60,000/year by her decision to change to multinutrients, it is unwilling to cover, or even subsidize, the cost of evidence-based supplements. Unfortunately, policy makers have not been open to examining this issue, despite repeated efforts to bring it to their attention.

Marie's perspective: the following statement was written by Marie, looking back on her mental health over the past twenty years:

I have survived an overwhelming and dangerous journey of treatment, only to discover that what I actually needed was to feed my brain and recognize I was having a normal reaction to trauma and stress. It may sound strange to some people, but the truth is that I am well because I did *not* do what my doctors told me. I did not accept their diagnoses, labels, opinions, or treatment, and there were many over the years. Ultimately, I did it my way and I'm alive because of it.

The important questions for me are these: (1) Why, when we know micronutrient therapy can help bring mental and emotional wellness, do we continue to ignore it in our system of health care? (2) Why, when we know the possibilities of healing with nutrition, and that it is safe and non-addictive, do we not choose this path of treatment *prior to* drugs that can be damaging and addictive?

Both questions boil down to the same thing: Why, within a so-called educated society and mental health care system, do we choose to invest in the most dangerous and expensive protocol first? This is the billion-dollar question.

Neither Andrew nor Marie currently needs any mental healthcare services. Both continue to use one of the broad-spectrum multinutrient formulas. They are saving our healthcare system a lot of money.

But the difference is that they pay for the nutrients themselves — anywhere from $50 to $100 per month — and there is still no government support for that. And we have come across far too many people who simply can't afford multinutrient supplements.

Just think of how much money could be saved if the treatment for even a fraction of people-in-need changed from $60,000/year to less than $1,200/year.

This stance is truly short-sighted. In Alberta, our healthcare costs constitute more than 40 percent of the provincial budget (that includes physical health too, but mental health care is rising the fastest). It is staggering to contemplate the potential savings to our tax dollars, yet reaching policy makers in Alberta has been completely impossible in spite of many, many efforts.

The Stigma of Mental Illness Will Be Eliminated

Bonnie recalls a time several years ago when the Canadian federal government threw millions of dollars into a nationwide campaign to generate new ideas to eliminate the stigma of mental illness. Of course, they were not interested in the nutrition research she had been publishing. But they should have been, because there is no stigma associated with needing to improve your diet! The stigma associated with mental health problems is usually generated by fear of the unknown. Not knowing what the cause of mental problems is — that's scary, because it means it could happen to you too.

The fastest way to eliminate the stigma of mental illness would be to return to the "diagnosis" used over a hundred years ago for people who exhibited mental symptoms — seeing them as a nutritional problem until proven otherwise. So in our vision of a Happier, Healthier Tomorrow, the emergence of mental health symptoms would be indicative of "imperfect nutrition."[6] And people will be taught how to eat better, *first*.

Positive Signs of Change

"Food insecurity" refers to not having enough money to buy the food you need. It is a huge problem all over the world, including in so-called developed countries. It is also a problem for young people, such as college students; food banks or food pantries are commonplace now on campuses. Some universities have community gardens. The University of California, San Francisco, created an app to let students know when food is left over from catered events, and some 69 percent of its student population — all postgraduates — immediately signed up. How well can they eat when food isn't donated? Christchurch, New Zealand (and likely other places, too), has developed a foraging app so that people can find fruit trees that are not on private land.

Wholesome Wave

Wholesome Wave, a nonprofit organization established in 2007 in Bridgeport, Connecticut, by James Beard award-winning chef Michel Nischan, increases the access and affordability of fresh fruits and vegetables for those in need. Through nutrition incentive programs such as the following two, Wholesome Wave enables food-insecure Americans to buy fresh fruits and vegetables, which in turn helps local farmers and boosts local economies:

- The SNAP (Supplemental Nutrition Assistance Program) Doubling program encourages people to spend their federal nutrition benefits at farmers' markets and community-supported agriculture groups, where they can receive $2 worth of locally grown, fresh produce for every $1 they spend in SNAP.

- Produce Prescriptions partners with local clinics and healthcare systems so that participants receive health and nutrition education. On average, each participant receives $1/day for purchase of fresh produce, which is more than some families currently spend on a per-person basis. These prescription programs also expose participants' taste buds to new kinds of veggies and fruits they might not have been able to afford before.

City Harvest in New York

Many efforts are being made in Western nations to salvage surplus food from stores and restaurants, and direct it toward those who are hungry. In New York City, a group called City Harvest (cityharvest.org) has been doing this important work since 1982. You can find something similar in almost every major city in the United States.

Nudge Interventions

Nudge interventions are methods of gently steering people toward better choices. Have you noticed that your school cafeteria has fresh fruit next to the cash register? That is a nudge intervention, based on the finding that many students get near the cash register and realize that they don't have enough food on their tray yet. They will grab whatever's closest, and an apple is a much better choice than a bag of potato chips.

It is a similar nudge rationale that led Berkeley, California, to pass the Healthy Checkout Ordinance that goes into effect March 2021. Large grocery stores will be required to have healthy food choices, and not ultra-processed items, within a three-foot radius of check-out counters.

A new nudge initiative has supermarkets in New Zealand giving away fruit for no cost as soon as customers walk in the door. It's a win/win. People love getting things for free. Since fresh fruit smells so good, if it encourages customers to buy more, the stores profit. And, of course, the customer's health improves the more fruit they eat. Some grocery stores in Canada do that, too, with free fruit designated for children.

In Europe, several countries have experimented with school-based programs, providing free fruit (and sometimes vegetables) at lunchtime to all children. Although the results are mixed, in general the availability of free fruit has resulted in increased consumption levels. For example, an evaluation of eight years of the Norwegian School Fruit Scheme for adolescents found approximately a 50 percent increase in fruit consumption.[7]

The Policy Changes We Need for a Healthier Tomorrow

Effective treatments with diet and nutrient supplements are being ignored in spite of ample scientific support because they do not fit the reigning dogma. The conventional medical model continues to emphasize "Treat with drugs first." Unfortunately, the drugs don't remove the disease and the patient often continues to struggle. Therefore, we have to reverse this perspective of "drugs first" with lifestyle changes like nutrition. These take longer, but will ultimately lead to health, not just the absence of some symptoms. Meds will then be able to take their more appropriate place as a *supplement.*

Our society continues to accept that mental health treatment can bring about only partial improvement rather than recovery. We prefer the slogan of the Foundation for Excellence in Mental Health Care (openexcellence.org): *Expect Recovery.*

It is realistic, and evidence-based, to demand the following seven policy changes from our governments and healthcare systems:

- Every expectant mother should be provided with accurate education on what to eat during pregnancy, including nutrient-dense food.
- Every child (especially) will be treated *first* with diet and then (if

needed) nutrients in pill form before ever exposing their developing brains to psychiatric medications.

- Every healthcare facility that deals with mental health will implement the educational content described in Step One in Our Vision, and ensure that every patient referred to their facility is offered the opportunity to learn about nutrition and the brain, and how to shop and cook.
- Every medical school will teach students the crucial role of nutrients in brain metabolism and mitochondrial function.
- Every psychiatric training program will educate its students about the potential of nutrition-related treatments.
- Every healthcare system will accommodate the cost of nutrition education, as well as the much less expensive option of treating with broad-spectrum multinutrient formulas rather than medications.
- Agribusiness will re-examine its widespread practice of sterilizing the earth's microbiome, and will help our food producers improve the mineral density of our soil.

Will fulfillment of these demands put psychiatrists out of business? Of course not. Many of them would welcome the opportunity of spending more time talking to their patients, helping them through life's difficult challenges. After all, that's mostly what has drawn people to specializing in psychiatry in the first place.

The Takeaway

Is our vision of a Happier, Healthier Tomorrow realistic? We think so! If we can just convince policy makers to pay attention to the fact that nutrition is key to building the Better Brain!

EPILOGUE

We Shouldn't Have to Wait 264 Years
for Better Brain Health!

The doctor of the future will no longer treat the human frame with drugs, but
rather will cure and prevent disease with nutrition.

— THOMAS EDISON (1847–1931)

The Scurvy Story

MOST PEOPLE KNOW THAT insufficient vitamin C causes scurvy, but
few people in the current era realize what a huge health problem it was
a few centuries ago.[1] In the fifteenth and sixteenth centuries, it was not
unusual for 40 percent of sailors on long voyages to die of scurvy. They
would become weak, their gums would bleed, their teeth would become
loose, their skin would bruise, and they were depressed. Death was often
unavoidable.

In 1601 a ship captain named James Lancaster decided to give the sailors on his ship three spoonfuls of bottled lemon juice every day, because
there was a suspicion that something in citrus (vitamins had not yet been
discovered) was making sailors healthier. The result: the men on the
other ships in his fleet were devastated by scurvy, but not on his.

A Scottish doctor named James Lind took the next step in 1747. When twelve sailors on his ship developed scurvy, he randomly assigned them to six groups of two each. They continued to eat the same food, but group one received a quart of cider daily, group two received a small amount of sulfuric acid, the third group was given six spoonfuls of vinegar, group four had to drink a half a pint of seawater, group five received two oranges and one lemon, and group six was given some barley water with a spicy paste. By the sixth day the ship ran out of fruit, but the two men in the citrus group (number five) had already recovered. The only others to benefit were in group one — the men drinking a quart of cider showed some improvement.

Wouldn't you think that the Lancaster and Lind trials would have resulted in an immediate policy change for all the British ships? You would be wrong.

It took the British Admiralty another forty-eight years before it required navy ships to carry citrus fruits. And that's not all. It took another seventy years for the British Board of Trade to require citrus on all merchant ships.

The time from scientific proof in 1601 to regulated practice in 1865 was a whopping 264 years!

What's the lesson here for mental health? Bonnie and her colleagues traced the scientific studies of minerals and vitamins to treat mental disorders back to the 1920s.[2] The earliest work was off-track, focusing on a single nutrient at a time. The research on B-complex vitamins to lessen medication doses was first published in 1992. Multinutrient treatment research really took off around 2000. Now we have RCT evidence of efficacy, cost savings, reduced side effects, and general health benefits.

That's a hundred years. After exactly a *century* of data accumulation, we all need to demand policy changes. How long will it take our society to recognize that suboptimal nutrition is contributing to the epidemic of mental disorders?

Answering the Age-Old Question:
What Causes Mental Illness?

Bonnie entitles some of her lectures to clinicians with a question: *Are we treating mental illness or nutrient deficiency?* As you've learned, many mental symptoms can be caused by suboptimal nutrition. But as you've also learned, we can't conclude that, for example, people who are depressed are not eating well. It is possible to eat an excellent whole foods diet and still be experiencing serious mental health challenges.

Some possible causes: 1) the foods themselves might not be nutrient-dense, 2) some people might have inherited a need for more minerals and vitamins to enable their brains to produce and break down all the neurotransmitters and other brain chemicals needed for optimal brain health, and 3) there are other complex genetic, family, and community stressors playing a major role in that person's life.

We still don't know the answer to this age-old question: What causes mental illness? We *do* know that, throughout history, lack of good nutrition has been high on the list of answers. And we also know that it has been neglected for about seventy years.

Nutrition was considered to be a major factor as recently as 1917 when the *People's Home Library* was published in America. The disappearance of nutrition from the mental health treatment list coincided with the psychopharmacology "revolution" that began in the United States in the 1960s. But even during the years in which we were told to just pop a pill to treat anxiety, depression, or just a crummy bad day, some very sharp minds continued to emphasize nutrients and brain function. These are the people who have fostered orthomolecular psychiatry, integrative medicine, and functional medicine. Conventional medicine continues to promote primarily pharmaceutical treatment.

The Three Societal Issues That We
Often Wonder About

For us, there are many questions that emerge from everything we have discussed in this book. When will conventional pharmaceutically influenced physicians begin to learn and appreciate nutrition for mental health? When will the public begin to understand that their diet affects their brain? We could go on. But for society as a whole, there are these three broad societal issues:

1. Can our health systems change in response to the new scientific evidence? Will our current system of funding and regulation be able to adapt to a Nutrition First approach to mental health? Will people be able to get help paying for scientifically supported nutrient treatments?

2. How do we help those people who don't want, or don't respond to, medications? Right now, a simple and inexpensive solution to mental health disorders is being ignored and disdained because it's "just" nutrition. We've lost count of how many people have told us that they got better, and that they could think more clearly and manage their stress better, when they changed their diet and/or started taking a broad-spectrum supplement. These anecdotes are supported by the controlled clinical trials you've read about in this book.

3. Why do our societies seem to readily accept data showing that nutrition and other lifestyle factors like exercise and quitting smoking are good for our *hearts,* but find it so hard to accept the use of diet and supplements to make us feel better *mentally*? With 20 percent of us suffering from mental disorders, it is long past time for change. Businesses are suffering from sick leave costs for mental health.

Schools and universities spend much of their scarce resources on mental health services. Children are given drugs when they're still very young, and no one knows what the long-term effects of these drugs do to developing brains.

We all need to understand that the social burden of poor food choices is too great. The stakes are just too high. It's imposing a big stress on our society as a whole.

Decades ago, when seemingly everyone smoked in restaurants, on airplanes, in glossy magazine ads, on TV shows and in movies, and even in doctors' offices, few would have believed that smoking would end up banned in public and private spaces, and even in cafés in Paris! If smoking can go from being perceived as "glamorous" to something that can kill you, then we can rethink our approach to mental health treatments, too.

Change is *not* difficult. Change *is* possible. Change *is* achievable.

ACKNOWLEDGMENTS

In scientific research, we always stand on the shoulders of giants. We thank the many pioneers for their perseverance, often in the face of unbelievable obstacles. Gene Arnold is an inspiring example, because he has steadfastly championed the importance of evaluating non-drug treatment options for children with ADHD and other mental challenges. The late Abram Hoffer is another example, as he withstood ostracism by his own professional association to pursue nutrient treatment for the benefit of his patients. We are so grateful to Charlie Popper for twenty years of guidance, wisdom, and friendship; his influence on us both has been vast. We especially thank Andrew Weil for his generous foreword to this book, and Victoria Maizes for first inviting us to bring our work to the attention of integrative physicians — and to both of them for their support and networking assistance, and most of all for committing their own energy to educating their medical colleagues about nutrition.

We cherish our other scientific collaborators who have faced many struggles with us: Neville Blampied, Mary Fristad, Dermot Gately, Barbara Gracious, Jeni Johnstone, Bryan Kolb (who first opened the door, and then pushed Bonnie through it), Brenda Leung, Lewis Mehl-Madrona, John Perham, Ian Shaw. And also all the other nutrition researchers around the world who have seen the importance of looking at the interface between nutrition and mental health.

We are especially indebted to the psychiatrists and other physicians who supported this research when nutrient therapy was a controversial idea, especially within their own profession: Anna Boggis, Larry Cormier, Matt Eggleston, Roger Mulder, Megan Rodway, Scott Shannon, Steve Simpson. Each of these individuals played a key role at a critical time, and our work benefited from their open minds.

We acknowledge with awe the vision and determination of Tony Stephan and the late David Hardy, and all their relatives and associates at Truehope Nutritional Support and Hardy Nutritionals, for knowing that there is nothing more important than changing the way mental health challenges are treated. For these families, making money has never been the issue. For all of them, the goal has been *tikkun olam* (repairing the world), a Hebrew expression Bonnie taught them in the 1990s.

Although we are fully responsible for any errors, we thank all the people who lent their expertise for fact checking and interpretations, especially: Jim Adams, John Cryan, Deb Dewey, Elissa Epel, Gerry Giesbrecht, Martin Kennedy, David Smith, and Mikki Williden.

We have so appreciated working with people, especially at Aevitas and HMH, who made our first book publishing experience relatively pain-free: Karen Moline (our collaborator who remarkably translated our scientific jargon into writing for the general public), Karen Murgolo and Laura Nolan (our agents, both of whom could see the big-picture vision and potential global impact of our work), and our editor, Sarah Pelz, who "got it" from the first time we spoke to her in 2019. We also thank Judith Choate (our recipe expert).

We thank our universities, the University of Calgary and the University of Canterbury, for giving us the environment and support to conduct our research.

We are so grateful to our donors who have enabled us to do the research described in this book, while maintaining our integrity to always be independently funded until the future when (we hope) governments begin to fund this line of research: Margaret Bailey (NZ), George Bass (US), the late Bob Church (Canada), the late Marie Lockie (NZ), Allan Markin (Canada), Cheryl Payer (US), Jake Plattner (US), Seymour Weingarten (US), and many more who have been donating to the two community foundations managing the charitable funds Bonnie established in 2015 to support young scientists studying nutritional treatments — the Foundation for Excellence in Mental Health Care (US) and the Calgary Foundation (Canada). We also thank the Vic Davis Memorial Trust (NZ), the GAMA Foundation (NZ), the Canterbury Medical Research Foundation (NZ), the University of Canterbury Foundation (NZ), the Christchurch Foundation (NZ), and the Waterloo Foundation (Wales).

From Bonnie

Many thanks to the agricultural nutrition experts who have shared their knowledge and listened to our data so that we all understand that what they do in the field is directly relevant to society's brain health: Harvey Dann, the late David Hardy, Don Huber, Dave Nelson, James Porterfield, and Howard Vlieger.

A special thanks to my husband, Richard, and son, Jonathan, and to all the friends whom I studiously ignored for at least ten years when they told me repeatedly that I had a unique perspective about mental health and really ought to write a book. I apologize to all of them for being slow to agree.

From Julia

A special acknowledgment to Kaila Colbin and the TEDx team, who invited me to the Christchurch TEDx stage, giving the public an evidence-based go-to video that has changed lives around the world.

Special thanks to my parents, who taught me to be curious and to stand up for what is right, no matter how much it might challenge the world-view; my three brothers and friends, who supported me throughout this journey of discovery; my two sons, Duncan and Toby, who have grown up amidst this transformational research; and my husband, Will, my rock.

Nā tō rourou, nā taku rourou, ka ora ai te iwi.

With your food basket and my food basket, the people will be healthy.

RESOURCES

From Introduction: Julia's 2014 TEDx talk

https://www.youtube.com/watch?v=3dqXHHCc5lA

From chapter 3: Information about regenerative agriculture

Soil Health Academy Schools (soilhealthacademy.org)
Acres USA (acresusa.com)
Rodale Institute (rodaleinstitute.org)
Savory Institute (savory.global)

From chapters 3, 10: Sources of information on pesticides, herbicides, the Dirty Dozen, and the Clean Fifteen

Environmental Working Group (ewg.org)

From chapter 5: Website devoted to new conversations about mental health

MadInAmerica.com

From chapter 6: A training video to help people learn to swallow pills and capsules

Research4kids.ucalgary.ca/pillswallowing

From chapter 8: The Healthy Eating Plate

https://www.health.harvard.edu/staying-healthy/healthy-eating-plate

From chapter 10: Dietary guidelines

Nutrition Coalition (nutritioncoalition.us)

http://www.fao.org/nutrition/education/food-dietary-guidelines/home/
en/

From chapter 11: Websites of the nutrient formulas mentioned

www.Truehope.com

www.HardyNutritionals.com

https://www.autismnrc.org

https://www.buyberocca.com/en/home/

http://www.blackmores.com.au/products/executive-b-stress-formula

https://swisse.com/

http://www.forceval.co.uk

https://www.enlyterx.com/

www.optimox.com

A full list of the research behind all of the multinutrient products described
can be found on the publications tab at TheBetterBrainBook.com.

From chapter 12: Groups working on improving access
to nutritious food in the United States

Wholesome Wave (wholesomewave.org)

City Harvest (cityharvest.org)

Imperfect Foods (imperfectfoods.com)

Julia recently developed an online course through edX (www.edx.org) on
nutrition and mental health. You can audit the course for free or get a
certificate by completing the assignments: https://www.edx.org/course/
mental-health-and-nutrition

A portion of the proceeds from the sale of this book will go toward
supporting future research on micronutrient treatment of mental health
problems. The three charitable funds established for this purpose are:
In the United States: the Nutrition and Mental Health Research Fund,

managed by the Foundation for Excellence in Mental Health Care
(openexcellence.org)

In Canada: the Nutrition and Mental Health Fund, managed by the Calgary
Foundation (CalgaryFoundation.org)

In New Zealand: the University of Canterbury Foundation (https://www
.canterbury.ac.nz/uc-foundation)

NOTES

Foreword

1. Stephen Devries, James Dalen, David Eisenberg, Victoria Maizes, et al., "A Deficiency of Nutrition Education in Medical Training," *American Journal of Medicine* 127, no. 9 (2014): 804–806.
2. Farin Kamangar and Ashkan Emadi, "Vitamin and Mineral Supplements: Do We Really Need Them?" *International Journal of Preventive Medicine* 3, no. 3 (2012): 221–26.
3. Andrew Weil, *Mind over Meds* (New York: Little, Brown, 2016).

Introduction

1. Thomas Moore and Donald Mattison, "Adult Utilization of Psychiatric Drugs and Differences by Sex, Age, and Race," *JAMA Internal Medicine* 177, no. 2 (2017): 274–75.
2. Jay Amsterdam, Leemon McHenry, and Jon Jureidini, "Industry-Corrupted Psychiatric Trials," *Psychiatria Polska* 51, no. 6 (2017): 993–1008.

1. The Missing Key for Mental Health

1. Devries, Dalen, Eisenberg, Maizes, et al., "A Deficiency of Nutrition Education."
2. Simran Maggo, Martin Kennedy, Zoe Barczyk, Allison Miller, et al., "Common CYP2D6, CYP2C9, and CYP2C19 Gene Variants, Health Anxiety, and Neuroticism Are Not Associated with Self-Reported Antidepressant Side Effects," *Frontiers in Genetics* 10, no. 1199 (2019): 1199.
3. Megan Rodway, Annette Vance, Amany Watters, Helen Lee, et al., "Efficacy and Cost of Micronutrient Treatment of Childhood Psychosis," *BMJ Case Reports* (2012): 10.1136/bcr-2012-007213.
4. Simon Kemp, *Medieval Psychology* (USA: Greenwood Press, 1990).
5. Thomas Ritter, *The People's Home Library* (USA: The R.C. Barnum Co., 1910).
6. Howard Brody, "Pharmaceutical Industry Financial Support for Medical Education: Benefit, or Undue Influence?" *Journal of Law, Medicine and Ethics* 37, no. 3 (2009): 451–60.
7. Bonnie Kaplan, Susan Crawford, Catherine Field, and Steven Simpson, "Vitamins, Minerals, and Mood," *Psychological Bulletin* 133, no. 5 (2007): 747–60.
8. Myrto Samara, Adriani Nikolakopoulou, Georgia Salanti, and Stefan Leucht, "How Many Patients with Schizophrenia Do Not Respond to Antipsychotic Drugs in the Short Term? An Analysis Based on Individual Patient Data from Randomized Controlled Trials," *Schizophrenia Bulletin* 45, no. 3 (2018): 639–46.
9. Joanna Moncrieff, "Are Antidepressants as Effective as Claimed? No, They Are Not Effective at

All," *Canadian Journal of Psychiatry* 52, no. 2 (2007): 96–97; Joanna Moncrieff, "Misrepresenting Harms in Antidepressant Trials," *BMJ* 352 (2016): i217.

10. David Healy and Chris Whitaker, "Antidepressants and Suicide: Risk-Benefit Conundrums," *Journal of Psychiatry and Neuroscience* 28, no. 5 (2003): 331–37; Tarang Sharma, Louise Guski, Nanna Freund, and Peter Gøtzsche, "Suicidality and Aggression During Antidepressant Treatment: Systematic Review and Meta-Analyses Based on Clinical Study Reports," *BMJ* 352 (2016): i65.

11. Michael Hengartner and Martin Plöderl, "Newer-Generation Antidepressants and Suicide Risk in Randomized Controlled Trials: A Re-Analysis of the FDA Database," *Psychotherapy and Psychosomatics* 88, no. 4 (2019): 247–48.

12. Peter Breggin and Ginger Breggin, *Talking Back to Prozac: What Doctors Aren't Telling You About Prozac and the Newer Antidepressants* (USA: Open Road Media, 2014).

13. Marc De Hert, Hendra Hudyana, Liesbeth Dockx, Chiara Bernagie, et al., "Second-Generation Antipsychotics and Constipation: A Review of the Literature," *European Psychiatry* 26, no. 1 (2011): 34–44.

14. John Read, Claire Cartwright, and Kerry Gibson, "Adverse Emotional and Interpersonal Effects Reported by 1829 New Zealanders While Taking Antidepressants," *Psychiatry Research* 216, no. 1 (2014): 67–73.

15. New Zealand Government, *He Ara Oranga: Report of the Government Inquiry into Mental Health and Addiction* (Wellington, New Zealand: New Zealand Government, 2018).

16. Lex Wunderink, Roeline Nieboer, Durk Wiersma, Sjoerd Sytema, et al., "Recovery in Remitted First-Episode Psychosis at 7 Years of Follow-up of an Early Dose Reduction/Discontinuation or Maintenance Treatment Strategy: Long-Term Follow-up of a 2-Year Randomized Clinical Trial," *JAMA Psychiatry* 70, no. 9 (2013): 913–20.

17. Michael Hengartner, James Davies, and John Read, "Antidepressant Withdrawal — the Tide Is Finally Turning," *Epidemiology and Psychiatric Sciences* 29 (2019): 1–3.

18. Miriam Larsen-Barr, Fred Seymour, John Read, and Kerry Gibson, "Attempting to Discontinue Antipsychotic Medication: Withdrawal Methods, Relapse and Success," *Psychiatry Research* 270 (2018): 365–74; Peter Groot and Jim van Os, "Outcome of Antidepressant Drug Discontinuation with Tapering Strips after 1–5 Years," *Therapeutic Advances in Psychopharmacology* 10 (2020).

19. Devries, Dalen, Eisenberg, Maizes, et al., "A Deficiency of Nutrition Education."

20. Christopher Murray, Charles Atkinson, Kavi Bhalla, Gretchen Birbeck, et al., "The State of US Health, 1990–2010: Burden of Diseases, Injuries, and Risk Factors," *JAMA* 310, no. 6 (2013): 591–608.

2. Food for Thought: The Nutrients Your Brain Needs

1. Carola Janssen and Amanda Kiliaan, "Long-Chain Polyunsaturated Fatty Acids (LCPUFA) from Genesis to Senescence: The Influence of LCPUFA on Neural Development, Aging, and Neurodegeneration," *Progress in Lipid Research* 53 (2014): 1–17.

2. John Fernstrom, "A Perspective on the Safety of Supplemental Tryptophan Based on Its Metabolic Fates," *Journal of Nutrition* 146, no. 12 (2016): 2601s–2608s.

3. Chantal Courtemanche, Arnold Huang, Ilan Elson-Schwab, Nicole Kerry, et al., "Folate Deficiency and Ionizing Radiation Cause DNA Breaks in Primary Human Lymphocytes: A Comparison," *FASEB Journal* 18, no. 1 (2004): 209–11.

4. Richard Border, Emma Johnson, Luke Evans, Andrew Smolen, et al., "No Support for Historical Candidate Gene or Candidate Gene-by-Interaction Hypotheses for Major Depression Across Multiple Large Samples," *American Journal of Psychiatry* 176, no. 5 (2019): 376–87.

5. Laramie Duncan, Michael Ostacher, and Jacob Ballon, "How Genome-Wide Association Studies (GWAS) Made Traditional Candidate Gene Studies Obsolete," *Neuropsychopharmacology* 44, no. 9 (2019): 1518–23.

6. Wenfu Mao, Mary Schuler, and May Berenbaum, "A Dietary Phytochemical Alters Caste-Associated Gene Expression in Honey Bees," *Science Advances* 1, no. 7 (2015): e1500795.

7. Dana Dolinoy, "The Agouti Mouse Model: An Epigenetic Biosensor for Nutritional and Environmental Alterations on the Fetal Epigenome," *Nutrition Reviews* 66, Suppl 1 (2008): S7–S11.

8. Honghuang Lin, Gail Rogers, Kathryn Lunetta, Daniel Levy, et al., "Healthy Diet Is Associated with Gene Expression in Blood: The Framingham Heart Study," *American Journal of Clinical Nutrition* 110, no. 3 (2019): 742–49.

9. Aaron Stevens, Julia Rucklidge, Kathryn Darling, Matthew Eggleston, et al., "Methylomic Changes in Response to Micronutrient Supplementation and MTHFR Genotype," *Epigenomics* 10, no. 9 (2018): 1201–14.

10. Bonnie Kaplan, Gerald Giesbrecht, Brenda Leung, Catherine Field, et al., "The Alberta Pregnancy Outcomes and Nutrition (APrON) Cohort Study: Rationale and Methods," *Maternal and Child Nutrition* 10, no. 1 (2014): 44–60.

11. Maede Ejaredar, Elias Nyanza, Kayla Ten Eycke, and Deborah Dewey, "Phthalate Exposure and Children's Neurodevelopment: A Systematic Review," *Environmental Research* 142 (2015): 51–60; Maede Ejaredar, Yoonshin Lee, Derek Roberts, Reginald Sauve, et al., "Bisphenol A Exposure and Children's Behavior: A Systematic Review," *Journal of Exposure Science & Environmental Epidemiology* 27, no. 2 (2017): 175–83.

12. Melody Grohs, Jess Reynolds, Jiaying Liu, Jonathan Martin, et al., "Prenatal Maternal and Childhood Bisphenol A Exposure and Brain Structure and Behavior of Young Children," *Environmental Health* 18, no. 1 (2019): 85.

13. Gerald Giesbrecht, Maede Ejaredar, Jiaying Liu, Jenna Thomas, et al., "Prenatal Bisphenol A Exposure and Dysregulation of Infant Hypothalamic-Pituitary-Adrenal Axis Function: Findings from the APrON Cohort Study," *Environmental Health* 16, no. 1 (2017): 47.

14. Gillian England-Mason, Melody Grohs, Jess Reynolds, Amy MacDonald, et al., "White Matter Microstructure Mediates the Association Between Prenatal Exposure to Phthalates and Behavior Problems in Preschool Children," *Environmental Research* 182 (2020): 109093.

15. Dana Dolinoy, Dale Huang, and Randy Jirtle, "Maternal Nutrient Supplementation Counteracts Bisphenol A-Induced DNA Hypomethylation in Early Development," *Proceedings of the National Academy of Sciences of the United States of America* 104, no. 32 (2007): 13056–61.

16. Bernhard Hennig, Lindell Ormsbee, Craig McClain, Bruce Watkins, et al., "Nutrition Can Modulate the Toxicity of Environmental Pollutants: Implications in Risk Assessment and Human Health," *Environmental Health Perspectives* 120, no. 6 (2012): 771–74.

17. Bruce Ames, Ilan Elson-Schwab, and Eli Silver, "High-Dose Vitamin Therapy Stimulates Variant Enzymes with Decreased Coenzyme Binding Affinity (Increased $K(M)$): Relevance to Genetic Disease and Polymorphisms," *American Journal of Clinical Nutrition* 75, no. 4 (2002): 616–58.

18. Julia Rucklidge, Matthew Eggleston, Kathryn Darling, Aaron Stevens, et al., "Can We Predict Treatment Response in Children with ADHD to a Vitamin-Mineral Supplement? An Investigation into Pre-Treatment Nutrient Serum Levels, MTHFR Status, Clinical Correlates and Demographic Variables," *Progress in Neuro-Psychopharmacology and Biological Psychiatry* 89 (2019): 181–92.

19. Bonnie Kaplan and Scott Shannon, "Nutritional Aspects of Child and Adolescent Psychopharmacology," *Pediatric Annals* 36, no. 9 (2007): 600–609.

20. Joseph Salami, Haider Warraich, Javier Valero-Elizondo, Erica Spatz, et al., "National Trends in Statin Use and Expenditures in the US Adult Population from 2002 to 2013: Insights from the Medical Expenditure Panel Survey," *JAMA Cardiology* 2, no. 1 (2017): 56–65.

21. Cristiana Berti, Hans Biesalski, Roland Gartner, Alexandre Lapillonne, et al., "Micronutrients in Pregnancy: Current Knowledge and Unresolved Questions," *Clinical Nutrition* 30, no. 6 (2011): 689–701.

22. Brenda Leung and Bonnie Kaplan, "Perinatal Depression: Prevalence, Risks, and the Nutrition Link — a Review of the Literature," *Journal of the American Dietetic Association* 109, no. 9 (2009): 1566–75.

23. Fariba Aghajafari, Catherine Field, Bonnie Kaplan, Doreen Rabi, et al., "The Current Recommended Vitamin D Intake Guideline for Diet and Supplements During Pregnancy Is Not Adequate to Achieve Vitamin D Sufficiency for Most Pregnant Women," *PloS One* 11, no. 7 (2016): e0157262.

24. Junxiu Liu, Colin Rehm, Jennifer Onopa, and Dariush Mozaffarian, "Trends in Diet Quality Among Youth in the United States, 1999–2016," *JAMA* 323, no. 12 (2020): 1161–74.

25. James Joseph, Barbara Shukitt-Hale, Natalie Denisova, Ronald Prior, et al., "Long-Term Dietary Strawberry, Spinach, or Vitamin E Supplementation Retards the Onset of Age-Related Neuronal Signal-Transduction and Cognitive Behavioral Deficits," *Journal of Neuroscience* 18, no. 19 (1998): 8047–55.

26. Ilianna Lourida, Eilis Hannon, Thomas Littlejohns, Kenneth Langa, et al., "Association of Lifestyle and Genetic Risk with Incidence of Dementia," *JAMA* 322, no. 5 (2019): 430–37.

27. Marshall Miller, Derek Hamilton, James Joseph, and Barbara Shukitt-Hale, "Dietary Blueberry Improves Cognition Among Older Adults in a Randomized, Double-Blind, Placebo-Controlled Trial," *European Journal of Nutrition* 57, no. 3 (2018): 1169–80.

28. Marta Crous-Bou, Teresa Fung, Jennifer Prescott, Bettina Julin, et al., "Mediterranean Diet and Telomere Length in Nurses' Health Study: Population Based Cohort Study," *BMJ* 349 (2014): g6674.

29. Lucia Alonso-Pedrero, Ana Ojeda-Rodríguez, Miguel Martínez-González, Guillermo Zalba, et al., "Ultra-Processed Food Consumption and the Risk of Short Telomeres in an Elderly Population of the Seguimiento Universidad de Navarra (Sun) Project," *American Journal of Clinical Nutrition* 111, no. 6 (2020): 1259–66.

30. Martha Morris, Christy Tangney, Yamin Wang, Frank Sacks, et al., "MIND Diet Associated with Reduced Incidence of Alzheimer's Disease," *Alzheimer's and Dementia* 11, no. 9 (2015): 1007–14.

31. Martha Morris, Christy Tangney, Yamin Wang, Frank Sacks, et al., "MIND Diet Slows Cognitive Decline with Aging," *Alzheimer's and Dementia* 11, no. 9 (2015): 1015–22.

32. Guangwen Tang, Catherine Serfaty-Lacrosniere, Maria Camilo, and Robert Russell, "Gastric Acidity Influences the Blood Response to a Beta-Carotene Dose in Humans," *American Journal of Clinical Nutrition* 64, no. 4 (1996): 622–26.

3. Not Your Grandmother's Peach: Factors That Have Led to Decreased Nutrient Intake

1. Ron Sender, Shai Fuchs, and Ron Milo, "Are We Really Vastly Outnumbered? Revisiting the Ratio of Bacterial to Host Cells in Humans," *Cell* 164, no. 3 (2016): 337–40.

2. John Cryan, Kenneth O'Riordan, Caitlin Cowan, Kiran Sandhu, et al., "The Microbiota-Gut-Brain Axis," *Physiological Reviews* 99, no. 4 (2019): 1877–2013.

3. Cryan, O'Riordan, Cowan, Sandhu, et al., "The Microbiota-Gut-Brain Axis."

4. Richard Frye, John Slattery, Derrick MacFabe, Emma Allen-Vercoe, et al., "Approaches to Studying and Manipulating the Enteric Microbiome to Improve Autism Symptoms," *Microbial Ecology in Health and Disease* 26 (2015): 26878.

5. Elaine Hsiao, Sara McBride, Sophia Hsien, Gil Sharon, et al., "Microbiota Modulate Behavioral and Physiological Abnormalities Associated with Neurodevelopmental Disorders," *Cell* 155, no. 7 (2013): 1451–63.

6. Stephen Collins, Zain Kassam, and Premysl Bercik, "The Adoptive Transfer of Behavioral Phenotype via the Intestinal Microbiota: Experimental Evidence and Clinical Implications," *Current Opinion in Microbiology* 16, no. 3 (2013): 240–45.

7. Collins, Kassam, and Bercik, "The Adoptive Transfer of Behavioral Phenotype."

8. Maria Cenit, Yolanda Sanz, and Pilar Codoner-Franch, "Influence of Gut Microbiota on Neuropsychiatric Disorders," *World Journal of Gastroenterology* 23, no. 30 (2017): 5486–98.

9. Sigrid Breit, Aleksandra Kupferberg, Gerhard Rogler, and Gregor Hasler, "Vagus Nerve as Modulator of the Brain-Gut Axis in Psychiatric and Inflammatory Disorders," *Frontiers in Psychiatry* 9 (2018): 44.

10. Thomas Bastiaanssen, Caitlin Cowan, Marcus Claesson, Timothy Dinan, et al., "Making Sense of . . . The Microbiome in Psychiatry," *International Journal of Neuropsychopharmacology* 22, no. 1 (2019): 37–52.

11. Karen-Anne McVey Neufeld, Pauline Luczynski, Clara Seira Oriach, Timothy Dinan, et al., "What's Bugging Your Teen? The Microbiota and Adolescent Mental Health," *Neuroscience and Biobehavioral Reviews* 70 (2016): 300–12.

12. Jessica Flannery, Keaton Stagaman, Adam Burns, Roxana Hickey, et al., "Gut Feelings Begin in Childhood: The Gut Metagenome Correlates with Early Environment, Caregiving, and Behavior," *mBio* 11, no. 1 (2020): e02780-19.

13. Cryan, O'Riordan, Cowan, Sandhu, et al., "The Microbiota-Gut-Brain Axis."

14. Mireia Valles-Colomer, Gwen Falony, Youssef Darzi, Ettje Tigchelaar, et al., "The Neuroactive Potential of the Human Gut Microbiota in Quality of Life and Depression," *Nature Microbiology* 4, no. 4 (2019): 623–32.

15. Erica Sonnenburg and Justin Sonnenburg, "Starving Our Microbial Self: The Deleterious Consequences of a Diet Deficient in Microbiota-Accessible Carbohydrates," *Cell Metabolism* 20, no. 5 (2014): 779–86.

16. Richard Liu, Rachel Walsh, and Ana Sheehan, "Prebiotics and Probiotics for Depression and Anxiety: A Systematic Review and Meta-Analysis of Controlled Clinical Trials," *Neuroscience and Biobehavior Reviews* 102 (2019): 13–23.

17. Asma Kazemi, Ahmad Noorbala, Kamal Azam, Mohammad Eskandari, et al., "Effect of Probiotic and Prebiotic vs Placebo on Psychological Outcomes in Patients with Major Depressive Disorder: A Randomized Clinical Trial," *Clinical Nutrition* 38, no. 2 (2018): 522–28.

18. Kirsten Tillisch, Jennifer Labus, Lisa Kilpatrick, Zhiguo Jiang, et al., "Consumption of Fermented Milk Product with Probiotic Modulates Brain Activity," *Gastroenterology* 144, no. 7 (2013): 1394-401.e4.

19. Qin Ng, Wayren Loke, Nandini Venkatanarayanan, Donovan Lim, et al., "A Systematic Review of the Role of Prebiotics and Probiotics in Autism Spectrum Disorders," *Medicina (Kaunas, Lithuania)* 55, no. 5 (2019); Richard Liu, Rachel Walsh, and Ana Sheehan, "Prebiotics and Probiotics for Depression and Anxiety: A Systematic Review and Meta-Analysis of Controlled Clinical Trials," *Neuroscience and Biobehavior Reviews* 102 (2019): 13–23; Elnaz Vaghef-Mehrabany, Vahid Maleki, Maryam Behrooz, Fatemeh Ranjbar, et al., "Can Psychobiotics 'Mood'ify Gut? An Update Systematic Review of Randomized Controlled Trials in Healthy and Clinical Subjects, on Anti-Depressant Effects of Probiotics, Prebiotics, and Synbiotics," *Clinical Nutrition* 39, no. 5 (2020): 1395–1410.

20. Timothy Dinan, Catherine Stanton, and John Cryan, "Psychobiotics: A Novel Class of Psychotropic," *Biological Psychiatry* 74, no. 10 (2013): 720–26.

21. Collins, Kassam, and Bercik, "The Adoptive Transfer of Behavioral Phenotype."

22. Anna Pärtty, Marko Kalliomäki, Pirjo Wacklin, Seppo Salminen, et al., "A Possible Link Between Early Probiotic Intervention and the Risk of Neuropsychiatric Disorders Later in Childhood: A Randomized Trial," *Pediatric Research* 77, no. 9 (2015): 823–28.

23. Faming Zhang, Bota Cui, Xingxiang He, Yuqiang Nie, et al., "Microbiota Transplantation: Concept, Methodology and Strategy for Its Modernization," *Protein Cell* 9 no. 5 (2018): 462–73.

24. Els van Nood, Anne Vrieze, Max Nieuwdorp, Susana Fuentes, et al., "Duodenal Infusion of Donor Feces for Recurrent Clostridium Difficile," *New England Journal of Medicine* 368, no. 5 (2013): 407–15.

25. Nicolien de Clercq, Myrthe Frissen, Mark Davids, Albert Groen, et al., "Weight Gain After Fecal Microbiota Transplantation in a Patient with Recurrent Underweight Following Clinical Recovery from Anorexia Nervosa," *Psychotherapy and Psychosomatics* 88, no. 1 (2019): 58–60.

26. Ting Cai, Xiao Shi, Ling-zhi Yuan, Dan Tang, et al., "Fecal Microbiota Transplantation in an Elderly Patient with Mental Depression," *International Psychogeriatrics* 31, no. 10 (2019): 1525–26.

27. Dae-Wook Kang, James Adams, Devon Coleman, Elena Pollard, et al., "Long-Term Benefit of Microbiota Transfer Therapy on Autism Symptoms and Gut Microbiota," *Scientific Reports* 9, no. 1 (2019): 5821; Dae-Wook Kang, James Adams, Ann Gregory, Thomas Borody, et al., "Microbiota Transfer Therapy Alters Gut Ecosystem and Improves Gastrointestinal and Autism Symptoms: An Open-Label Study," *Microbiome* 5, no. 1 (2017): 10.

28. Shunya Kurokawa, Taishiro Kishimoto, Shinta Mizuno, Tatsuhiro Masaoka, et al., "The Effect of Fecal Microbiota Transplantation on Psychiatric Symptoms Among Patients with Irritable Bowel Syndrome, Functional Diarrhea and Functional Constipation: An Open-Label Observational Study," *Journal of Affective Disorders* 235 (2018): 506–12.

29. Aaron Stevens, Rachel Purcell, Kathryn Darling, Matthew Eggleston, et al., "Human Gut Microbiome Changes During a 10 Week Randomised Control Trial for Micronutrient Supplementation in Children with Attention Deficit Hyperactivity Disorder," *Scientific Reports* 9, no. 1 (2019): 10128.

30. Cryan, O'Riordan, Cowan, Sandhu, et al., "The Microbiota-Gut-Brain Axis."

31. Robin Marles, "Mineral Nutrient Composition of Vegetables, Fruits and Grains: The Context of Reports of Apparent Historical Declines," *Journal of Food Composition and Analysis* 56 (2017): 93–103.

32. Adriana Martinez and Abraham Al-Ahmad, "Effects of Glyphosate and Aminomethylphosphonic Acid on an Isogeneic Model of the Human Blood-Brain Barrier," *Toxicology Letters* 304 (2019): 39–49.

33. Alexis Temkin and Olga Naidenko, "Glyphosate Contamination in Food Goes Far Beyond Oat Products," Science Review, *Environmental Working Group News and Analysis*, February 28, 2019.

34. Luiz Zobiole, Rubem Oliveira, Jesui Visentainer, Robert Kremer, et al., "Glyphosate Affects Seed Composition in Glyphosate-Resistant Soybean," *Journal of Agricultural and Food Chemistry* 58, no. 7 (2010): 4517–22.

35. Robin Mesnage, Maxime Teixeira, Daniele Mandrioli, Laura Falcioni, et al., "Shotgun Metagenomics and Metabolomics Reveal Glyphosate Alters the Gut Microbiome of Sprague-Dawley Rats by Inhibiting the Shikimate Pathway," *bioRxiv* (2019): 870105.

36. Ariena Van Bruggen, Miaomiao He, Keumchul Shin, Volker Mai, et al., "Environmental and Health Effects of the Herbicide Glyphosate," *Science of the Total Environment* 616–17 (2018): 255–68.

37. Judy Carman, Howard Vlieger, Larry Ver Steeg, Vertyn Sneller, et al., "A Long-Term Toxicology Study on Pigs Fed a Combined Genetically Modified (Gm) Soy and Gm Maize Diet," *Journal of Organic Systems* 8, no. 38–54 (2013).

38. Anthony Samsel and Stephanie Seneff, "Glyphosate, Pathways to Modern Diseases II: Celiac Sprue and Gluten Intolerance," *Interdisciplinary Toxicology* 6, no. 4 (2013): 159–84.

39. Carmen, Vlieger, Ver Steeg, Sneller, et al., "A Long-Term Toxicology Study on Pigs,"; Samsel and Seneff, "Glyphosate, Pathways to Modern Diseases."

40. John Fagan, Larry Bohlen, Sharyle Patton, and Kendra Klein, "Organic Diet Intervention Significantly Reduces Urinary Glyphosate Levels in U.S. Children and Adults," *Environmental Research* 189 (2020).

41. Samuel Myers and Matthew Smith, "Impact of Anthropogenic CO_2 Emissions on Global Human Nutrition," *Nature Climate Change* 8 (2018).

42. Petra Hogy, Herbert Wieser, Peter Kohler, Klaus Schwadorf, et al., "Effects of Elevated CO_2 on Grain Yield and Quality of Wheat: Results from a 3-Year Free-Air CO_2 Enrichment Experiment," *Plant Biology* 11, Suppl 1 (2009): 60–69.

4. The Power of the Food You Eat

1.   Felice Jacka, Julie Pasco, Arnstein Mykletun, Lana Williams, et al., "Association of Western and Traditional Diets with Depression and Anxiety in Women," *American Journal of Psychiatry* 167, no. 3 (2010): 305–11.

2.   Kyoung Kim, Myung Lim, Ho-Jang Kwon, Seung-Jin Yoo, et al., "Associations Between Attention-Deficit/Hyperactivity Disorder Symptoms and Dietary Habits in Elementary School Children," *Appetite* 127 (2018): 274–79.

3.   Kate Brookie, Georgia Best, and Tamlin Conner, "Intake of Raw Fruits and Vegetables Is Associated with Better Mental Health Than Intake of Processed Fruits and Vegetables," *Frontiers in Psychology* 9 (2018): 487.

4.   John Ekwaru, Arto Ohinmaa, Sarah Loehr, Solmaz Setayeshgar, et al., "The Economic Burden of Inadequate Consumption of Vegetables and Fruit in Canada," *Public Health Nutrition* 20, no. 3 (2017): 515–23.

5.   Ashima Kant, "Reported Consumption of Low-Nutrient-Density Foods by American Children and Adolescents: Nutritional and Health Correlates, Nhanes III, 1988 to 1994," *Archives of Pediatrics and Adolescent Medicine* 157, no. 8 (2003): 789–96.

6.   Jennifer Poti, Michelle Mendez, Shu Ng, and Barry Popkin, "Is the Degree of Food Processing and Convenience Linked with the Nutritional Quality of Foods Purchased by US Households?" *American Journal of Clinical Nutrition* 101, no. 6 (2015): 1251–62.

7.   Seung Lee-Kwan, Latetia Moore, Heidi Blanck, Diane Harris, et al., "Disparities in State-Specific Adult Fruit and Vegetable Consumption — United States, 2015," *Morbidity and Mortality Weekly Report* 66, no. 45 (2017): 1241–47.

8.   Jean-Claude Moubarac, M. Batal, M. Louzada, Martinez Steele, et al., "Consumption of Ultra-Processed Foods Predicts Diet Quality in Canada," *Appetite* 108 (2017): 512–20.

9.   Karen Davison, Lovedeep Gondara, and Bonnie Kaplan, "Food Insecurity, Poor Diet Quality, and Suboptimal Intakes of Folate and Iron Are Independently Associated with Perceived Mental Health in Canadian Adults," *Nutrients* 9, no. 3 (2017): 274.

10. Joseph Hibbeln and Rachel Gow, "The Potential for Military Diets to Reduce Depression, Suicide, and Impulsive Aggression: A Review of Current Evidence for Omega-3 and Omega-6 Fatty Acids," *Military Medicine* 179, no. 11 (2014): 117–28.

11. Tasnime Akbaraly, Eric Brunner, Jane Ferrie, Michael Marmot, et al., "Dietary Pattern and Depressive Symptoms in Middle Age," *British Journal of Psychiatry* 195, no. 5 (2009): 408–13.

12. Almudena Sánchez-Villegas, Estefania Toledo, Jokin de Irala, Miguel Ruiz-Canela, et al., "Fast-Food and Commercial Baked Goods Consumption and the Risk of Depression," *Public Health Nutrition* 15, no. 3 (2012): 424–32.

13. Olivia Loewen, Katerina Maximova, John Ekwaru, Erin Faught, et al., "Lifestyle Behavior and Mental Health in Early Adolescence," *Pediatrics* 143, no. 5 (2019).

14. Olivia Loewen, Katerina Maximova, John Ekwaru, Mark Asbridge, et al., "Adherence to Life-Style Recommendations and Attention-Deficit/Hyperactivity Disorder: A Population-Based Study of Children Aged 10 to 11 Years," *Psychosomatic Medicine* 82, no. 3 (2020): 305–15.

15. Felice Jacka, Peter Kremer, Michael Berk, Andrea de Silva-Sanigorski, et al., "A Prospective Study of Diet Quality and Mental Health in Adolescents," *PLoS One* 6, no. 9 (2011): e24805.

16. Erin Hoare, Meghan Hockey, Anu Ruusunen, and Felice Jacka, "Does Fruit and Vegetable Consumption During Adolescence Predict Adult Depression? A Longitudinal Study of US Adolescents," *Frontiers in Psychiatry* 9, no. 581 (2018).

17. Akiko Nanri, Tetsuya Mizoue, Kalpana Poudel-Tandukar, Mitsuhiko Noda, et al., "Dietary Patterns and Suicide in Japanese Adults: The Japan Public Health Center-Based Prospective Study," *British Journal of Psychiatry* 203, no. 6 (2013): 422–27.

18. Colin Mathers and Dejan Loncar, "Projections of Global Mortality and Burden of Disease from 2002 to 2030," *PLoS Medicine* 3, no. 11 (2006): e442.

19. Rachel Baskin, Briony Hill, Felice Jacka, Adrienne O'Neil, et al., "The Association Between

Diet Quality and Mental Health During the Perinatal Period: A Systematic Review," *Appetite* 91 (2015): 41–47.

20. Alan Brown and Ezra Susser, "Prenatal Nutritional Deficiency and Risk of Adult Schizophrenia," *Schizophrenia Bulletin* 34, no. 6 (2008): 1054–63; Changwei Li, Toni Miles, Luqi Shen, Ye Shen, et al., "Early-Life Exposure to Severe Famine and Subsequent Risk of Depressive Symptoms in Late Adulthood: The China Health and Retirement Longitudinal Study," *British Journal of Psychiatry* 213, no. 4 (2018): 579–86.

21. Felice Jacka, Elvind Ystrom, Anne Brantsaeter, Evalill Karevold, et al., "Maternal and Early Postnatal Nutrition and Mental Health of Offspring by Age 5 Years: A Prospective Cohort Study," *Journal of the American Academy of Child and Adolescent Psychiatry* 52, no. 10 (2013): 1038–47.

22. Cedric Galera, Barbara Heude, Anne Forhan, Jonathan Bernard, et al., "Prenatal Diet and Children's Trajectories of Hyperactivity-Inattention and Conduct Problems from 3 to 8 Years: The Eden Mother-Child Cohort," *Journal of Child Psychology and Psychiatry and Allied Disciplines* 59, no. 9 (2018): 1003–11.

23. Jolien Steenweg-de Graaff, Henning Tiemeier, Regine Steegers-Theunissen, Albert Hofman, et al., "Maternal Dietary Patterns During Pregnancy and Child Internalising and Externalising Problems: The Generation R Study," *Clinical Nutrition* 33, no. 1 (2014): 115–21.

24. Francois Bolduc, Amanda Lau, Cory Rosenfelt, Steven Langer, et al., "Cognitive Enhancement in Infants Associated with Increased Maternal Fruit Intake During Pregnancy: Results from a Birth Cohort Study with Validation in an Animal Model," *EBioMedicine* 8 (2016): 331–40.

25. Joseph Hibbeln, Steven Gregory, Yasmin Iles-Caven, Caroline Taylor, et al., "Total Mercury Exposure in Early Pregnancy Has No Adverse Association with Scholastic Ability of the Offspring Particularly If the Mother Eats Fish," *Environment International* 116 (2018): 108–15.

26. Jeffrey Mattes and Rachel Gittelman, "Effects of Artificial Food Colorings in Children with Hyperactive Symptoms: A Critical Review and Results of a Controlled Study," *Archives of General Psychiatry* 38, no. 6 (1981): 714–18.

27. Bonnie Kaplan, Jane McNicol, Richard Conte, and Hamid Moghadam, "Dietary Replacement in Preschool-Aged Hyperactive Boys," *Pediatrics* 83, no. 1 (1989): 7–17.

28. Joel Nigg, Kara Lewis, Tracy Edinger, and Michael Falk, "Meta-Analysis of Attention-Deficit/Hyperactivity Disorder or Attention-Deficit/Hyperactivity Disorder Symptoms, Restriction Diet, and Synthetic Food Color Additives," *Journal of the American Academy of Child and Adolescent Psychiatry* 51, no. 1 (2012): 86–97.

29. Nigg, Lewis, Edinger, and Falk, "Meta-Analysis of Attention-Deficit/Hyperactivity Disorder."

30. Felice Jacka, Adrienne O'Neil, Rachelle Opie, Catherine Itsiopoulos, et al., "A Randomised Controlled Trial of Dietary Improvement for Adults with Major Depression (the 'Smiles' Trial)," *BMC Medicine* 15, no. 1 (2017): 23.

31. Natalie Parletta, Dorota Zarnowiecki, Jihyun Cho, Amy Wilson, et al., "A Mediterranean-Style Dietary Intervention Supplemented with Fish Oil Improves Diet Quality and Mental Health in People with Depression: A Randomized Controlled Trial (HELFIMED)," *Nutritional Neuroscience* 22, no. 7 (2017): 1–14.

32. Heather Francis, Richard Stevenson, Jaime Chambers, Dolly Gupta, et al., "A Brief Diet Intervention Can Reduce Symptoms of Depression in Young Adults — a Randomised Controlled Trial," *PloS One* 14, no. 10 (2019): e0222768.

33. Tamlin Conner, Kate Brookie, Anitra Carr, Louise Mainvil, et al., "Let Them Eat Fruit! The Effect of Fruit and Vegetable Consumption on Psychological Well-Being in Young Adults: A Randomized Controlled Trial," *PloS One* 12, no. 2 (2017): e0171206.

34. Jeni Fisk, Sundus Khalid, Shirley Reynolds, and Claire Williams, "Effect of 4 Weeks Daily Wild Blueberry Supplementation on Symptoms of Depression in Adolescents," *British Journal of Nutrition* 124, no. 2 (2020): 181–88.

35. Alan Kazdin, "Addressing the Treatment Gap: A Key Challenge for Extending Evidence-Based Psychosocial Interventions," *Behaviour Research and Therapy* 88 (2017): 7–18.

36. Jacqui Wise, "Only Half of Patients Referred for Talking Therapies Enter Treatment," *British Medical Journal* 348 (2014): 295.

5. Treating Psychiatric Disorders with Supplements

1. Julia Rucklidge, Christopher Frampton, Brigette Gorman, and Anna Boggis, "Vitamin-Mineral Treatment of Attention-Deficit Hyperactivity Disorder in Adults: Double-Blind Randomised Placebo-Controlled Trial," *British Journal of Psychiatry* 204, no. 4 (2014): 306–15.

2. Julia Rucklidge, Matthew Eggleston, Jeanette Johnstone, Kathryn Darling, et al., "Vitamin-Mineral Treatment Improves Aggression and Emotional Regulation in Children with ADHD: A Fully Blinded, Randomized, Placebo-Controlled Trial," *Journal of Child Psychology and Psychiatry and Allied Disciplines* 59, no. 3 (2018): 232–46.

3. Julia Rucklidge, Christopher Frampton, Brigette Gorman, and Anna Boggis, "Vitamin-Mineral Treatment of ADHD in Adults: A 1-Year Naturalistic Follow-up of a Randomized Controlled Trial," *Journal of Attention Disorders* 21, no. 6 (2017): 522–32; Kathryn Darling, Matthew Eggleston, Hāna Retallick-Brown, and Julia Rucklidge, "Mineral-Vitamin Treatment Associated with Remission in Attention-Deficit/Hyperactivity Disorder Symptoms and Related Problems: 1-Year Naturalistic Outcomes of a 10-Week Randomized Placebo-Controlled Trial," *Journal of Child and Adolescent Psychopharmacology* 29, no. 9 (2019): 688–704.

4. Jeanette Johnstone, Brenda Leung, Barbara Gracious, Leanna Perez, et al., "Rationale and Design of an International Randomized Placebo-Controlled Trial of a 36-Ingredient Micronutrient Supplement for Children with ADHD and Irritable Mood: The Micronutrients for ADHD in Youth (MADDY) Study," *Contemporary Clinical Trials Communications* 16 (2019): 100478.

5. James Adams and Charles Holloway, "Pilot Study of a Moderate Dose Multivitamin/Mineral Supplement for Children with Autism Spectrum Disorder," *Journal of Alternative and Complementary Medicine* 10, no. 6 (2004): 1033–39.

6. James Adams, Tapan Audhya, Sharon McDonough-Means, Robert Rubin, et al., "Effect of a Vitamin/Mineral Supplement on Children and Adults with Autism," *BMC Pediatrics* 11 (2011): 111.

7. James Adams, Tapan Audhya, Elizabeth Geis, Eva Gehn, et al., "Comprehensive Nutritional and Dietary Intervention for Autism Spectrum Disorder — a Randomized, Controlled 12-Month Trial," *Nutrients* 10, no. 3 (2018): 369.

8. Lewis Mehl-Madrona, Brenda Leung, Carla Kennedy, Sarah Paul, et al., "A Naturalistic Case-Control Study of Micronutrients Versus Standard Medication Management in Autism," *Journal of Child and Adolescent Psychopharmacology* 20, no. 2 (2010): 95–103.

9. Bonnie Kaplan, Steven Simpson, Richard Ferre, Chris Gorman, et al., "Effective Mood Stabilization with a Chelated Mineral Supplement: An Open-Label Trial in Bipolar Disorder," *Journal of Clinical Psychiatry* 62, no. 12 (2001): 936–44; Charles Popper, "Do Vitamins or Minerals (Apart from Lithium) Have Mood-Stabilising Effects?" *Journal of Clinical Psychiatry* 62, no. 12 (2001): 933–35; Miles Simmons, "Nutritional Approach to Bipolar Disorder," *Journal of Clinical Psychiatry* 64, no. 3 (2003): 338; Elisabeth Frazier, Barbara Gracious, Eugene Arnold, Mark Failla, et al., "Nutritional and Safety Outcomes from an Open-Label Micronutrient Intervention for Pediatric Bipolar Spectrum Disorders," *Journal of Child and Adolescent Psychopharmacology* 23, no. 8 (2013): 558–67; Bonnie Kaplan, Paula Hilbert, and Ekaterina Tsatsko, "Micronutrient Treatment for Children with Emotional and Behavioral Dysregulation: A Case Series," *Journal of Medical Case Reports* 9 (2015): 240.

10. Bonnie Kaplan, Susan Crawford, Beryl Gardner, and Geraldine Farrelly, "Treatment of Mood Lability and Explosive Rage with Minerals and Vitamins: Two Case Studies in Children," *Journal of Child and Adolescent Psychopharmacology* 12, no. 3 (2002): 205–19.

11. Dermot Gately and Bonnie Kaplan, "Database Analysis of Adults with Bipolar Disorder Consuming a Multinutrient Formula," *Clinical Medicine: Psychiatry* 4 (2009): 3–16.

12. Julia Rucklidge, Dermot Gately, and Bonnie Kaplan, "Database Analysis of Children and Adolescents with Bipolar Disorder Consuming a Micronutrient Formula," *BMC Psychiatry* 10, no. 1 (2010): 74.

13. Kaplan, Crawford, Gardner, and Farrelly, "Treatment of Mood Lability and Explosive Rage."

14. Mariska Bot, Ingeborg Brouwer, Miquel Roca, Elisabeth Kohls, et al., "Effect of Multinutrient Supplementation and Food-Related Behavioral Activation Therapy on Prevention of Major Depressive Disorder Among Overweight or Obese Adults with Subsyndromal Depressive Symptoms: The MooDFOOD Randomized Clinical Trial," *JAMA* 321, no. 9 (2019): 858–68.

15. Arnold Mech and Andrew Farah, "Correlation of Clinical Response with Homocysteine Reduction During Therapy with Reduced B Vitamins in Patients with MDD Who Are Positive for MTHFR C677T or A1298C Polymorphism: A Randomized, Double-Blind, Placebo-Controlled Study," *Journal of Clinical Psychiatry* 77, no. 5 (2016): 668–71.

16. Jerome Sarris, Gerard Byrne, Con Stough, Chad Bousman, et al., "Nutraceuticals for Major Depressive Disorder — More Is Not Merrier: An 8-Week Double-Blind, Randomised, Controlled Trial," *Journal of Affective Disorders* 245 (2019): 1007–15.

17. Michael Berk, Alyna Turner, Gin Malhi, Chee Ng, et al., "A Randomised Controlled Trial of a Mitochondrial Therapeutic Target for Bipolar Depression: Mitochondrial Agents, N-Acetylcysteine, and Placebo," *BMC Medicine* 17, no. 1 (2019): 18.

18. Samantha Kimball, Naghmeh Mirhosseini, and Julia Rucklidge, "Database Analysis of Depression and Anxiety in a Community Sample-Response to a Micronutrient Intervention," *Nutrients* 10, no. 2 (2018).

19. Meredith Blampied, Caroline Bell, Claire Gilbert, Joseph Boden, et al., "Study Protocol for a Randomized Double Blind, Placebo Controlled Trial Exploring the Effectiveness of a Micronutrient Formula in Improving Symptoms of Anxiety and Depression," *Medicines* 5, no. 2 (2018): 56.

20. Phuong Nguyen, Ann DiGirolamo, Ines Gonzalez-Casanova, Hoa Pham, et al., "Impact of Preconceptional Micronutrient Supplementation on Maternal Mental Health During Pregnancy and Postpartum: Results from a Randomized Controlled Trial in Vietnam," *BMC Women's Health* 17, no. 1 (2017): 44.

21. Anna Paoletti, Marisa Orru, Maria Marotto, Monica Pilloni, et al., "Observational Study on the Efficacy of the Supplementation with a Preparation with Several Minerals and Vitamins in Improving Mood and Behaviour of Healthy Puerperal Women," *Gynecological Endocrinology* 29, no. 8 (2013): 779–83.

22. Rebecca Schmidt, Ana-Maria Iosif, Elizabeth Guerrero Angel, and Sally Ozonoff, "Association of Maternal Prenatal Vitamin Use with Risk for Autism Spectrum Disorder Recurrence in Young Siblings," *JAMA Psychiatry* 76, no. 4 (2019): 391–98; Jasveer Virk, Zeyan Liew, Jørn Olsen, Ellen Nohr, et al., "Pre-Conceptual and Prenatal Supplementary Folic Acid and Multivitamin Intake, Behavioral Problems, and Hyperkinetic Disorders: A Study Based on the Danish National Birth Cohort (DNBC)," *Nutritional Neuroscience* 21, no. 5 (2017): 1–9.

23. Anna Vinkhuyzen, Darryl Eyles, Thomas Burne, Laura Blanken, et al., "Gestational Vitamin D Deficiency and Autism Spectrum Disorder," *BJPsych Open* 3, no. 2 (2017): 85–90.

24. Robert Freedman, Sharon Hunter, and Camille Hoffman, "Prenatal Primary Prevention of Mental Illness by Micronutrient Supplements in Pregnancy," *American Journal of Psychiatry* 175, no. 7 (2018): 607–19.

25. Hayley Bradley, Siobhan Campbell, Roger Mulder, Jacki Henderson, et al., "Can Micronutrients Treat Symptoms of Antenatal Depression and Anxiety and Impact Infant Development? Study Protocol for the Efficacy and Safety of a Double Blind, Randomized, Placebo Controlled Trial (the 'NUTRIMUM' Trial)," *BMC Pregnancy and Childbirth* 20, no. 1 (2020): 488.

26. Lewis Mehl-Madrona and Barbara Mainguy, "Adjunctive Treatment of Psychotic Disorders with Micronutrients," *Journal of Alternative and Complementary Medicine* 23, no. 7 (2017): 526–33.

6. Tackling Life's Challenges with Supplements

1. Rachel Harrison, Julia Rucklidge, and Neville Blampied, "Use of Micronutrients Attenuates Cannabis and Nicotine Abuse as Evidenced from a Reversal Design: A Case Study," *Journal of Psychoactive Drugs* 45, no. 2 (2013): 1–11.

2. Phillipa Reihana, Neville Blampied, and Julia Rucklidge, "Novel Mineral-Vitamin Treatment for Reduction in Cigarette Smoking: A Fully Blinded Randomized Placebo-Controlled Trial," *Nicotine and Tobacco Research* 21, no. 11 (2018): 1496–505.

3. Bonnie Kaplan, Jennifer Fisher, Susan Crawford, Catherine Field, et al., "Improved Mood and Behavior During Treatment with a Mineral-Vitamin Supplement: An Open-Label Case Series of Children," *Journal of Child and Adolescent Psychopharmacology* 14, no. 1 (2004): 115–22; Bonnie Kaplan and Brenda Leung, "Multi-Micronutrient Supplementation for the Treatment of Psychiatric Symptoms," *Integrative Medicine: A Clinician's Journal* 10, no. 3 (2011); Julia Rucklidge, Matthew Eggleston, Jeanette Johnstone, Kathryn Darling, et al., "Vitamin-Mineral Treatment Improves Aggression and Emotional Regulation in Children with ADHD: A Fully Blinded, Randomized, Placebo-Controlled Trial," *Journal of Child Psychology and Psychiatry and Allied Disciplines* 59, no. 3 (2018): 232–46.

4. David Fraser, "Mineral-Deficient Diets and the Pig's Attraction to Blood: Implications for Tail-Biting," *Canadian Journal of Animal Science* 67, no. 4 (1987): 909–18.

5. Stephen Schoenthaler, Stephen Amos, Walter Doraz, Mary-Ann Kelly, et al., "The Effect of Randomized Vitamin-Mineral Supplementation on Violent and Non-Violent Antisocial Behavior Among Incarcerated Juveniles," *Journal of Nutritional and Environmental Medicine* 7 (1997): 343–52.

6. Stephen Schoenthaler and Ian Bier, "The Effect of Vitamin-Mineral Supplementation on Juvenile Delinquency Among American Schoolchildren: A Randomized, Double-Blind Placebo-Controlled Trial," *Journal of Alternative and Complementary Medicine* 6, no. 1 (2000): 7–17.

7. Ap Zaalberg, Henk Nijman, Erik Bulten, Luwe Stroosma, et al., "Effects of Nutritional Supplements on Aggression, Rule-Breaking, and Psychopathology Among Young Adult Prisoners," *Aggressive Behavior* 36, no. 2 (2010): 117–26; Bernard Gesch, Sean Hammond, Sarah Hampson, Aanita Eves, et al., "Influence of Supplementary Vitamins, Minerals and Essential Fatty Acids on the Antisocial Behaviour of Young Adult Prisoners," *British Journal of Psychiatry* 181 (2002): 22–28.

8. Ans Eilander, Tarun Gera, Harshpal Sachdev, Catherine Transler, et al., "Multiple Micronutrient Supplementation for Improving Cognitive Performance in Children: Systematic Review of Randomized Controlled Trials," *American Journal of Clinical Nutrition* 91, no. 1 (2010): 115–30.

9. David Kennedy and Crystal Haskell, "Vitamins and Cognition: What Is the Evidence?" *Drugs* 71, no. 15 (2011): 1957–71.

10. David Smith, Helga Refsum, Teodoro Bottiglieri, Michael Fenech, et al., "Homocysteine and Dementia: An International Consensus Statement," *Journal of Alzheimer's Disease* 62, no. 2 (2018): 561–70.

11. Gwenaelle Douaud, Helga Refsum, Celeste de Jager, Robin Jacoby, et al., "Preventing Alzheimer's Disease-Related Gray Matter Atrophy by B-Vitamin Treatment," *Proceedings of the National Academy of Sciences of the United States of America* 110, no. 23 (2013): 9523–28.

12. Smith, Refsum, Bottiglieri, Fenech, et al., "Homocysteine and Dementia."

13. Bonnie Kaplan, Caroline Leaney, and Ekatarina Tsatsko, "Micronutrient Treatment of Emotional Dyscontrol Following Traumatic Brain Injury," *Annals of Psychiatry and Mental Health* 4, no. 5 (2016): 1078.

14. Bryan Kolb, Celeste Halliwell, and Robbin Gibb, "Nutritional and Environmental Influences on Brain Development: Critical Periods of Brain Development, Pathways, and Mechanisms of Effect," in *Nutrition and the Developing Brain,* edited by Victoria Moran and Nicola Lowe (London: CRC Press, 2016).

15. R. London, L. Bradley, and N. Chiamori, "Effect of a Nutritional Supplement on Premenstrual Symptomatology in Women with Premenstrual Syndrome: A Double-Blind Longitudinal Study," *Journal of the American College of Nutrition* 10, no. 5 (1991): 494–99; Zaren Chakmakjian, C. E. Higgins, and G. E. Abraham, "The Effect of a Nutritional Supplement, Optivite for Women, on Premenstrual Tension Syndromes. II. Effect on Symptomatology, Using a Double Blind Cross-over Design," *Journal of Applied Nutrition* 37, no. 1 (1985): 12–17.

16. Katrina Wyatt, Paul Dimmock, Peter Jones, and Shaughn O'Brien, "Efficacy of Vitamin B-6 in the Treatment of Premenstrual Syndrome: Systematic Review," *British Medical Journal* 318, no. 7195 (1999): 1375–81.

17. Hāna Retallick-Brown, Neville Blampied, and Julia Rucklidge, "A Pilot Randomized Treatment-Controlled Trial Comparing Vitamin B6 with Broad-Spectrum Micronutrients for Premenstrual Syndrome," *Journal of Alternative and Complementary Medicine* 26, no. 2 (2020): 88–97.

18. Joanna Lothian, Neville Blampied, and Julia Rucklidge, "Effect of Micronutrients on Insomnia in Adults: A Multiple-Baseline Study," *Clinical Psychological Science* 4, no. 6 (2016): 1112–24.

7. Improving Resilience to Trauma and Stress with Supplements

1. Ronald Kessler, Maria Petukhova, Nancy Sampson, Alan Zaslavsky, et al., "Twelve-Month and Lifetime Prevalence and Lifetime Morbid Risk of Anxiety and Mood Disorders in the United States," *International Journal of Methods in Psychiatric Research* 21, no. 3 (2012): 169–84.

2. Sandra Galea, Arijit Nandi, and David Vlahov, "The Epidemiology of Post-Traumatic Stress Disorder After Disasters," *Epidemiologic Reviews* 27 (2005): 78–91.

3. Sandro Galea, Raina Merchant, and Nicole Lurie, "The Mental Health Consequences of Covid-19 and Physical Distancing: The Need for Prevention and Early Intervention," *JAMA Internal Medicine* 180, no. 6 (2020): 817–18.

4. Joanne Ingram, Greg Maciejewski, and Christopher Hand, "Changes in Diet, Sleep, and Physical Activity Are Associated with Differences in Negative Mood During COVID-19 Lockdown," *Frontiers in Psychology* 11, no. 2328 (2020).

5. Lauren Young, Andrew Pipingas, David White, Sarah Gauci, et al., "A Systematic Review and Meta-Analysis of B Vitamin Supplementation on Depressive Symptoms, Anxiety, and Stress: Effects on Healthy and 'at-Risk' Individuals," *Nutrients* 11, no. 9 (2019): 2232.

6. Julia Rucklidge, Jeanette Johnstone, Rachel Harrison, and Anna Boggis, "Micronutrients Reduce Stress and Anxiety in Adults with Attention-Deficit/Hyperactivity Disorder Following a 7.1 Earthquake," *Psychiatry Research* 189, no. 2 (2011): 281–87.

7. Douglas Carroll, Christopher Ring, Martin Suter, and Gonneke Willemsen, "The Effects of an Oral Multivitamin Combination with Calcium, Magnesium, and Zinc on Psychological Well-Being in Healthy Young Male Volunteers: A Double-Blind Placebo-Controlled Trial," *Psychopharmacology* 150, no. 2 (2000): 220–25; Lourens Schlebusch, Brenda Bosch, Graeme Polglase, I. Kleinschmidt, et al., "A Double-Blind, Placebo-Controlled, Double-Centre Study of the Effects of an Oral Multivitamin-Mineral Combination on Stress," *South African Medical Journal* 90, no. 12 (2000): 1216–23; David Kennedy, Rachel Veasey, Anthony Watson, Fiona Dodd, et al., "Effects of High-Dose B Vitamin Complex with Vitamin C and Minerals on Subjective Mood and Performance in Healthy Males," *Psychopharmacology* 211, no. 1 (2010): 55–68.

8. Julia Rucklidge, Rebecca Andridge, Brigette Gorman, Neville Blampied, et al., "Shaken but Unstirred? Effects of Micronutrients on Stress and Trauma After an Earthquake: RCT Evidence Comparing Formulas and Doses," *Human Psychopharmacology: Clinical and Experimental* 27, no. 5 (2012): 440–54.

9. Bonnie Kaplan, Julia Rucklidge, Amy Romijn, and Michael Dolph, "A Randomized Trial of Nutrient Supplements to Minimize Psychological Stress After a Natural Disaster," *Psychiatry Research* 228 (2015): 373–79.

10. Shahram Moosavi, Bernard Nwaka, Idowu Akinjise, Sandra Corbett, et al., "Mental Health

Effects in Primary Care Patients 18 Months After a Major Wildfire in Fort McMurray: Risk Increased by Social Demographic Issues, Clinical Antecedents, and Degree of Fire Exposure," *Frontiers in Psychiatry* 10 (2019): 683.

11. Julia Rucklidge, Usman Afzali, Bonnie Kaplan, Oindrila Bhattacharya et al., "Massacre, Earthquake, Flood: Translational Science Evidence that the Use of Micronutrients Post-disaster Reduces the Risk of Post-traumatic Stress in Survivors of Disasters," *International Perspectives in Psychology: Research, Practice, Consultation* (in press).

8. Food First: Eating Well, Mediterranean Style

1. Laura LaChance and Drew Ramsey, "Antidepressant Foods: An Evidence-Based Nutrient Profiling System for Depression," *World Journal of Psychiatry* 8, no. 3 (2018): 97–104.

2. Patrizia Ciminiello and Ernesto Fattorusso, "Bivalve Molluscs as Vectors of Marine Biotoxins Involved in Seafood Poisoning," *Progress in Molecular and Subcellular Biology* 43 (2006): 53–82.

3. Christine Pennesi and Laura Klein, "Effectiveness of the Gluten-Free, Casein-Free Diet for Children Diagnosed with Autism Spectrum Disorder: Based on Parental Report," *Nutritional Neuroscience* 15, no. 2 (2012): 85–91.

4. Jennifer Elder, Meena Shankar, Jonathan Shuster, Douglas Theriaque, et al., "The Gluten-Free, Casein-Free Diet in Autism: Results of a Preliminary Double Blind Clinical Trial," *Journal of Autism and Developmental Disorders* 36, no. 3 (2006): 413–20.

5. Faezeh Ghalichi, Jamal Ghaemmaghami, Ayyoub Malek, and Alireza Ostadrahimi, "Effect of Gluten Free Diet on Gastrointestinal and Behavioral Indices for Children with Autism Spectrum Disorders: A Randomized Clinical Trial," *World Journal of Pediatrics* 12, no. 4 (2016): 436–42.

6. Brunetta Porcelli, Verdino Verdino, Letizia Bossini, Lucia Terzuoli, et al., "Celiac and Non-Celiac Gluten Sensitivity: A Review on the Association with Schizophrenia and Mood Disorders," *Auto-Immunity Highlights* 5, no. 2 (2014): 55–61.

7. Stacey Bell, Gregory Grochoski, and Andrew Clarke, "Health Implications of Milk Containing Beta-Casein with the A2 Genetic Variant," *Critical Reviews in Food Science and Nutrition* 46, no. 1 (2006): 93–100.

8. Bonnie Beezhold, Carol Johnston, and Deanna Daigle, "Vegetarian Diets Are Associated with Healthy Mood States: A Cross-Sectional Study in Seventh Day Adventist Adults," *Nutrition Journal* 9 (2010): 26; Ulka Agarwal, Suruchi Mishra, Jia Xu, Susan Levin, et al., "A Multicenter Randomized Controlled Trial of a Nutrition Intervention Program in a Multiethnic Adult Population in the Corporate Setting Reduces Depression and Anxiety and Improves Quality of Life: The Geico Study," *American Journal of Health Promotion* 29, no. 4 (2015): 245–54.

9. Johannes Michalak, Xiao Zhang, and Frank Jacobi, "Vegetarian Diet and Mental Disorders: Results from a Representative Community Survey," *International Journal of Behavioral Nutrition and Physical Activity* 9 (2012): 67; Joseph Hibbeln, Kate Northstone, Jonathan Evans, and Jean Golding, "Vegetarian Diets and Depressive Symptoms Among Men," *Journal of Affective Disorders* 225 (2018): 13–17; Xiu-de Li, Hong-jong Cao, Shao-yu Xie, Kai-chun Li, et al., "Adhering to a Vegetarian Diet May Create a Greater Risk of Depressive Symptoms in the Elderly Male Chinese Population," *Journal of Affective Disorders* 243 (2019): 182–87.

10. Julie Pasco, Lana Williams, Neil Mann, Allison Hodge, et al., "Red Meat Consumption and Mood and Anxiety Disorders," *Psychotherapy and Psychosomatics* 81, no. 3 (2012): 196–98.

11. Giorgia Sebastiani, Ana Herranz Barbero, Cristina Borras-Novell, Miguel Alsina Casanova, et al., "The Effects of Vegetarian and Vegan Diet During Pregnancy on the Health of Mothers and Offspring," *Nutrients* 11, no. 3 (2019).

12. Roman Pawlak, Scott Parrott, Sudha Raj, Diana Cullum-Dugan, et al., "How Prevalent Is Vitamin B(12) Deficiency Among Vegetarians?" *Nutrition Reviews* 71, no. 2 (2013): 110–17.

13. Elisa Brietzke, Rodrigo Mansur, Mehala Subramaniapillai, Vicent Balanza-Martinez, et al., "Ketogenic Diet as a Metabolic Therapy for Mood Disorders: Evidence and Developments," *Neuroscience and Biobehavioral Reviews* 94 (2018): 11–16.

14. Cavin Balaster, *How to Feed a Brain: Nutrition for Optimal Brain Function and Repair* (Austin, TX: Feed a Brain LLC, 2017).

15. Margaret Defeyter and Riccardo Russo, "The Effect of Breakfast Cereal Consumption on Adolescents' Cognitive Performance and Mood," *Frontiers in Human Neuroscience* 7 (2013): 789.

16. Katie Adolphus, Clare Lawton, and Louise Dye, "The Effects of Breakfast on Behavior and Academic Performance in Children and Adolescents," *Frontiers in Human Neuroscience* 7 (2013): 425.

17. Rosario Ferrer-Cascales, Miriam Sánchez-SanSegundo, Nicolás Ruiz-Robledillo, Natalia Albaladejo-Blázquez, et al., "Eat or Skip Breakfast? The Important Role of Breakfast Quality for Health-Related Quality of Life, Stress and Depression in Spanish Adolescents," *International Journal of Environmental Research and Public Health* 15, no. 8 (2018).

18. Rachelle Opie, Adrienne O'Neil, Felice Jacka, Josephine Pizzinga, et al., "A Modified Mediterranean Dietary Intervention for Adults with Major Depression: Dietary Protocol and Feasibility Data from the Smiles Trial," *Nutritional Neuroscience* 21, no. 7 (2018): 487–501.

19. Rachelle Opie, Leonie Segal, Felice Jacka, Laura Nicholls, et al., "Assessing Healthy Diet Affordability in a Cohort with Major Depressive Disorder," *Journal of Public Health and Epidemiology* 7, no. 5 (2015): 159–69.

10. Foods to Avoid for a Better Brain

1. Stephen Schoenthaler, "The Effect of Sugar on the Treatment and Control of Antisocial Behavior: A Double-Blind Study of an Incarcerated Juvenile Population," *International Journal of Biosocial Research* 3, no. 1 (1982): 1–9.

2. Sara Mostafalou and Mohammad Abdollahi, "The Link of Organophosphorus Pesticides with Neurodegenerative and Neurodevelopmental Diseases Based on Evidence and Mechanisms," *Toxicology* 409 (2018): 44–52.

3. Ian Shaw, "Chemical Residues, Food Additives and Natural Toxicants in Food — the Cocktail Effect," *International Journal of Food Science & Technology* 49, no. 10 (2014): 2149–57.

11. Supplements: What You Need to Know

1. Julia Rucklidge, Jeanette Johnstone, Brigette Gorman, Anna Boggis, et al., "Moderators of Treatment Response in Adults with ADHD Treated with a Vitamin-Mineral Supplement," *Progress in Neuro-Psychopharmacology and Biological Psychiatry* 50 (2014): 163–71; Julia Rucklidge, Matthew Eggleston, Kathryn Darling, Aaron Stevens, et al., "Can We Predict Treatment Response in Children with ADHD to a Vitamin-Mineral Supplement? An Investigation into Pre-Treatment Nutrient Serum Levels, MTHFR Status, Clinical Correlates and Demographic Variables," *Progress in Neuro-Psychopharmacology and Biological Psychiatry* 89 (2019): 181–92.

2. Kiki van der Burg, Lachlan Cribb, Joseph Firth, Diana Karmacoska, et al., "Nutrient and Genetic Biomarkers of Nutraceutical Treatment Response in Mood and Psychotic Disorders: A Systematic Review," *Nutritional Neuroscience* (2019): 1–17.

3. Julia Rucklidge, Matthew Eggleston, Anna Boggis, Kathryn Darling, et al., "Do Changes in Blood Nutrient Levels Mediate Treatment Response in Children and Adults with ADHD Consuming a Vitamin–Mineral Supplement?" *Journal of Attention Disorders* (2020).

4. Julia Rucklidge, "Could Yeast Infections Impair Recovery from Mental Illness? A Case Study Using Micronutrients and Olive Leaf Extract for the Treatment of ADHD and Depression," *Advances in Mind-Body Medicine* 27, no. 3 (2013): 14–18.

5. Elisabeth Landaas, Tore Aarsland, Arve Ulvik, Anne Halmøy, et al., "Vitamin Levels in Adults with ADHD," *BJPsych Open* 2, no. 6 (2016): 377–84.

6. Maaike Bruins, Gladys Mugambi, Janneke Verkaik-Kloosterman, Jeljer Hoekstra, et al., "Addressing the Risk of Inadequate and Excessive Micronutrient Intakes: Traditional Versus New Approaches to Setting Adequate and Safe Micronutrient Levels in Foods," *Food and Nutrition Research* 59, no. 1 (2015): 26020.

7. Julia Rucklidge, Amy Harris, and Ian Shaw, "Are the Amounts of Vitamins in Commercially Available Dietary Supplement Formulations Relevant for the Management of Psychiatric Disorders in Children?" *New Zealand Medical Journal* 127, no. 1392 (2014): 73–85.

8. Popper, "Do Vitamins or Minerals (Apart from Lithium) Have Mood-Stabilising Effects?"

9. Con Stough, Andrew Scholey, Jenny Lloyd, Jo Spong, et al., "The Effect of 90 Day Administration of a High Dose Vitamin B-Complex on Work Stress," *Human Psychopharmacology* 26, no. 7 (2011): 470–76.

10. Jerome Sarris, Katherine Cox, David Camfield, Andrew Scholey, et al., "Participant Experiences from Chronic Administration of a Multivitamin Versus Placebo on Subjective Health and Wellbeing: A Double-Blind Qualitative Analysis of a Randomised Controlled Trial," *Nutrition Journal* 11, no. 1 (2012): 110; Elizabeth Harris, Joni Kirk, Renee Rowsell, Luis Vitetta, et al., "The Effect of Multivitamin Supplementation on Mood and Stress in Healthy Older Men," *Human Psychopharmacology* 26, no. 8 (2011): 560–67.

11. Ta-Wei Guu, David Mischoulon, Jerome Sarris, Joseph Hibbeln, et al., "International Society for Nutritional Psychiatry Research Practice Guidelines for Omega-3 Fatty Acids in the Treatment of Major Depressive Disorder," *Psychotherapy and Psychosomatics* 88, no. 5 (2019): 263–73.

12. Anthony Vesco, Andrea Young, Eugene Arnold, and Mary Fristad, "Omega-3 Supplementation Associated with Improved Parent-Rated Executive Function in Youth with Mood Disorders: Secondary Analyses of the Omega-3 and Therapy (OATS) Trials," *Journal of Child Psychology and Psychiatry, and Allied Disciplines* 59, no. 6 (2018): 628–36.

13. Jane Chang, Kuan-Pin Su, Valeria Mondelli, and Carmine Pariante, "Omega-3 Polyunsaturated Fatty Acids in Youths with Attention Deficit Hyperactivity Disorder: A Systematic Review and Meta-Analysis of Clinical Trials and Biological Studies," *Neuropsychopharmacology* 43, no. 3 (2018): 534–45.

14. Julia Rucklidge and Ian Shaw, "Are Over-the-Counter Fish Oil Supplements Safe, Effective and Accurate with Labelling? Analysis of 10 New Zealand Fish Oil Supplements," *New Zealand Medical Journal* 133, no. 1522 (2020): 52-62.

15. Rucklidge and Shaw, "Are Over-the-Counter Fish Oil Supplements Safe?"

16. Jason Lazarou, Bruce Pomeranz, and Paul Corey, "Incidence of Adverse Drug Reactions in Hospitalized Patients: A Meta-Analysis of Prospective Studies," *JAMA* 279, no. 15 (1998): 1200–1205.

17. Aristotle Voineskos, Benoit Mulsant, Erin Dickie, Nicholas Neufeld, et al., "Effects of Antipsychotic Medication on Brain Structure in Patients with Major Depressive Disorder and Psychotic Features: Neuroimaging Findings in the Context of a Randomized Placebo-Controlled Clinical Trial," *JAMA Psychiatry* 77, no. 7 (2020): 674–83.

18. Sanna Huhtaniska, Erika Jaaskelainen, Noora Hirvonen, Jukka Remes, et al., "Long-Term Antipsychotic Use and Brain Changes in Schizophrenia — a Systematic Review and Meta-Analysis," *Human Psychopharmacology* 32, no. 2 (2017): e2574.

19. David Gummin, James Mowry, Daniel Spyker, Daniel Brooks, et al., "2017 Annual Report of the American Association of Poison Control Centers' National Poison Data System (NPDS): 35th Annual Report," *Clinical Toxicology* (2018): 1–203.

20. Nadia Borlase, Tracy Melzer, Matthew Eggleston, Kathryn Darling, et al., "Resting-State Networks and Neurometabolites in Children with ADHD after 10 Weeks of Treatment with Micronutrients: Results of a Randomised Placebo-Controlled Trial," *Nutritional Neuroscience* (2019): 1–11; Stevens, Purcell, Darling, Eggleston, et al., "Human Gut Microbiome Changes"; Stevens, Rucklidge, Darling, Eggleston, et al., "Methylomic Changes in Response to Micronutrient Supplementation."

21. Brody, "Pharmaceutical Industry Financial Support."

22. Tarang Sharma, Louise Schow Guski, Nanna Freund, Dina Muscat Meng, et al., "Drop-out Rates in Placebo-Controlled Trials of Antidepressant Drugs: A Systematic Review and Meta-

Analysis Based on Clinical Study Reports," *International Journal of Risk & Safety in Medicine* 30, no. 4 (2019): 217–32.

23. Kolb, Halliwell, and Gibb, "Nutritional and Environmental Influences on Brain Development."

24. Steven Simpson, Susan Crawford, Estelle Goldstein, Catherine Field, et al., "Systematic Review of Safety and Tolerability of a Complex Micronutrient Formula Used in Mental Health," *BMC Psychiatry* 11 (2011): 62.

25. Adams, Audhya, Geis, Gehn, et al., "Comprehensive Nutritional and Dietary Intervention for Autism Spectrum Disorder."

26. Julia Rucklidge, Matthew Eggleston, Bre Ealam, Ben Beaglehole, et al., "An Observational Preliminary Study on the Safety of Long-Term Consumption of Micronutrients for the Treatment of Psychiatric Symptoms," *Journal of Alternative and Complementary Medicine* 25, no. 6 (2019): 613–22.

27. Irving Kirsch, Tania Huedo-Medina, H. Edmund Pigott, and Blair Johnson, "Do Outcomes of Clinical Trials Resemble Those 'Real World' Patients? A Reanalysis of the STAR*D Antidepressant Data Set," *Psychology of Consciousness: Theory, Research, and Practice* 5, no. 4 (2018): 339–45.

28. Rucklidge, Eggleston, Ealam, Beaglehole, et al., "An Observational Preliminary Study."

29. Goran Bjelakovic, Dimitrinka Nikolova, Lise Gluud, Rosa Simonetti, et al., "Antioxidant Supplements for Prevention of Mortality in Healthy Participants and Patients with Various Diseases," *Cochrane Database of Systematic Reviews*, no. 2 (2008): CD007176.

30. Hans Biesalski, Tilman Grune, Jana Tinz, Iris Zöllner, et al., "Reexamination of a Meta-Analysis of the Effect of Antioxidant Supplementation on Mortality and Health in Randomized Trials," *Nutrients* 2, no. 9 (2010): 929–49.

31. Iris Bell, Joel Edman, Frank Morrow, David Marby, et al., "Vitamin B1, B2, and B6 Augmentation of Tricyclic Antidepressant Treatment in Geriatric Depression with Cognitive Dysfunction," *Journal of the American College of Nutrition* 11, no. 2 (1992): 159–63; Jerome Sarris, David Mischoulon, and Isaac Schweitzer, "Adjunctive Nutraceuticals with Standard Pharmacotherapies in Bipolar Disorder: A Systematic Review of Clinical Trials," *Bipolar Disorders* 13, no. 5–6 (2011): 454–65; Nayereh Khoraminya, Medhi Tehrani-Doost, Shima Jazayeri, Aghafateme Hosseini, et al., "Therapeutic Effects of Vitamin D as Adjunctive Therapy to Fluoxetine in Patients with Major Depressive Disorder," *Australian and New Zealand Journal of Psychiatry* 47, no. 3 (2013): 271–75.

32. Charles Popper, "Single-Micronutrient and Broad-Spectrum Micronutrient Approaches for Treating Mood Disorders in Youth and Adults," *Child and Adolescent Psychiatric Clinics of North America* 23, no. 3 (2014): 591–672.

33. Bell, Edman, Morrow, Marby, et al., "Vitamin B1, B2, and B6 Augmentation of Tricyclic Antidepressant Treatment"; Khoraminya, Tehrani-Doost, Jazayeri, Hosseini, et al., "Therapeutic Effects of Vitamin D."

34. Popper, "Do Vitamins or Minerals (Apart from Lithium) Have Mood-Stabilising Effects?" Charles Popper, Bonnie Kaplan, and Julia Rucklidge, "Single and Broad-Spectrum Micronutrient Treatments in Psychiatry Practice," in *Complementary and Integrative Treatments in Psychiatric Practice*, edited by Patricia Gerbarg, Philip Muskin, and Richard Brown (Arlington: American Psychiatric Association Publishing, 2017), 75–104.

35. Gately and Kaplan, "Database Analysis of Adults with Bipolar Disorder Consuming a Multinutrient Formula."

36. Rucklidge, Gately, and Kaplan, "Database Analysis of Children and Adolescents with Bipolar Disorder Consuming a Micronutrient Formula."

37. David Bailey, George Dresser, and Malcolm Arnold, "Grapefruit-Medication Interactions: Forbidden Fruit or Avoidable Consequences?" *Canadian Medical Association Journal* 185, no. 4 (2013): 309–16.

38. Kavita Pandey, Suresh Naik, and Babu Vakil, "Probiotics, Prebiotics and Synbiotics — a Review," *Journal of Food Science and Technology* 52, no. 12 (2015): 7577–87.

12. A Vision for a Happier, Healthier Tomorrow

1. Eliseo Guallar, Saverio Stranges, Cynthia Mulrow, Lawrence Appel, et al., "Enough Is Enough: Stop Wasting Money on Vitamin and Mineral Supplements," *Annals of Internal Medicine* 159, no. 12 (2013): 850–51.
2. Mary Garcia-Cazarin, Edwina Wambogo, Karen Regan, and Cindy Davis, "Dietary Supplement Research Portfolio at the NIH, 2009–2011," *Journal of Nutrition* 144, no. 4 (2014): 414–18.
3. Ami Fukunaga, Yosuke Inoue, Takeshi Kochi, Huanhuan Hu, et al., "Prospective Study on the Association Between Adherence to Healthy Lifestyles and Depressive Symptoms Among Japanese Employees: The Furukawa Nutrition and Health Study," *Journal of Epidemiology* (2019).
4. Devries, Dalen, Eisenberg, Maizes, et al., "A Deficiency of Nutrition Education in Medical Training."
5. Bonnie Kaplan, Wanrudee Isaranuwatchai, and Jeffrey Hoch, "Hospitalization Cost of Conventional Psychiatric Care Compared to Broad-Spectrum Micronutrient Treatment: Literature Review and Case Study of Adult Psychosis," *International Journal of Mental Health Systems* 11 (2017): 14.
6. Ritter, *The People's Home Library.*
7. Ingrid Hovdenak, Elling Bere, and Tonje Stea, "Time Trends (1995–2008) in Dietary Habits Among Adolescents in Relation to the Norwegian School Fruit Scheme: The Hunt Study," *Nutrition Journal* 18, no. 1 (2019): 77.

Epilogue

1. Donald Berwick, "Disseminating Innovations in Health Care," *Journal of the American Medical Association* 289, no. 15 (2003): 1969–75.
2. Kaplan, Crawford, Field, and Simpson, "Vitamins, Minerals, and Mood."

INDEX

ABOUT THE AUTHORS

BONNIE J. KAPLAN, PhD, is a professor emerita in the Cumming School of Medicine at the University of Calgary, in Calgary, Alberta, Canada. Originally from Ohio, she did all her training in the United States (an honors baccalaureate degree in psychology at the University of Chicago, and master's and PhD degrees in experimental and physiological psychology at Brandeis University). Her interest in the biological basis of behavior led to postdoctoral training and then faculty research in neurophysiology at Yale University Department of Neurology and the West Haven (CT) Veterans Administration Neuropsychology Laboratory until she moved to Canada and the University of Calgary in 1979. She has published widely on the biological basis of developmental disorders and mental health, especially the contribution of nutrition to brain development and brain function. She was the founding principal investigator of the Alberta Pregnancy Outcomes and Nutrition Study (ApronStudy.ca). She is also a member of the International Society for Nutritional Psychiatry Research (ISNPR.org), which includes scientists studying the inflammatory basis of mental disorders, and the role of dietary intake. Bonnie has over 180 peer-reviewed publications and textbook contributions, and many more invited lectures. In 2018, for Canada's 150th birthday, she was named one of the country's top 150 Difference Makers in Mental Health. In 2019, she was awarded the prestigious Dr. Rogers Prize, a national award given every two years in Canada for research or clinical work in complementary, alternative, integrative health (drrogersprize.org). To learn more, visit: BonnieJKaplan.com

JULIA J. RUCKLIDGE, PhD, is a professor of clinical psychology in the School of Psychology, Speech, and Hearing at the University of Canterbury, Christchurch, New Zealand. Originally from Toronto, Ontario, Canada, she did her undergraduate training in neurobiology at McGill University in Montreal, and her master's and PhD at the University of Calgary in clinical psychology, followed by a two-year postdoctoral fellowship at the Hospital for Sick Children in Toronto. While in Alberta during her PhD studies, she first learned of people with mental illness benefiting from micronutrients. In 2000, she immigrated to New Zealand to take up her current position, and teaches child clinical psychology as well as a course devoted to mental health and nutrition, the only one of its kind in New Zealand. Over the last decade, her Mental Health and Nutrition Research Lab, *Te Puna Toiora,* has been running clinical trials investigating the role of broad-spectrum multinutrients in the treatment of mental illness, specifically ADHD, mood disorders, smoking, anxiety, and stress associated with traumatic events, including earthquakes, floods, and mass shootings. Julia has over 140 peer-reviewed publications and textbook contributions. She is regularly featured across social media, newspaper, radio, and television, and has given over 100 invited talks across the world on her work on nutrition and mental health. She is currently on the executive committee for the International Society of Nutritional Psychiatry Research (ISNPR.org), and a consultant on a multicentered EU-funded medical consortium studying the effects of nutrition on brain health (Eat-2beNICE). She was named one of the top 100 Most Influential Women in New Zealand in both 2015 and 2018 and received the Ballin award in 2015 from the New Zealand Psychological Society for her service to clinical psychology. Her 2014 TEDx talk has been viewed over 1.6 million times. Stay in touch on Facebook: www.facebook.com/mentalhealthan dnutrition, Twitter: @JuliaRucklidge, Instagram: www.instagram.com/ ucmentalhealthandnutrition, and visit her website to learn more: https:// www.canterbury.ac.nz/science/contact-us/people/julia-rucklidge.html

They were both featured in the documentary *Letters from Generation Rx,* directed by Kevin Miller and narrated by Tilda Swinton, that graphically displays the downside of our current treatment for mental illness.